THE
BEAUTY
PRESCRIPTION

◆

THE COMPLETE FORMULA FOR
LOOKING AND FEELING BEAUTIFUL

◆

Debra Luftman, M.D. & Eva Ritvo, M.D.

3 1336 08077 5316

New York   Chicago   San Francisco   Lisbon   London   Madrid   Mexico City
Milan   New Delhi   San Juan   Seoul   Singapore   Sydney   Toronto

The McGraw·Hill Companies

Library of Congress Cataloging-in-Publication Data

Luftman, Debra.
  The beauty prescription : the complete formula for looking and feeling
beautiful / by Debra Luftman and Eva Ritvo.
    p.   cm.
    ISBN 13: 978-0-07-154763-5 (alk. paper)
    ISBN 10: 0-07-154763-0 (alk. paper)
    1. Beauty, Personal.   2. Cosmetics.   3. Skin—Care and hygiene.
  I. Ritvo, Eva C., 1961–.   II. Title.

  RA776.98.L84   2009
  646.7′2—dc22   2008000362

1 2 3 4 5 6 7 8 9 10 11 12 13 14 15 16 17 18 19 20 21 22   FGR/FGR   0 9 8

ISBN   978-0-07-154763-5
MHID   0-07-154763-0

Interior design by DesignforBooks

McGraw-Hill books are available at special quantity discounts to use as premiums and
sales promotions or for use in corporate training programs. To contact a representative,
please visit the Contact Us pages at www.mhprofessional.com.

Maintaining patient confidentiality is paramount to the authors' integrity as health-care
professionals. This book is filled with anecdotes that resemble actual patient stories.
They are not. Each patient description is a fabrication based on composites shaped
from years of clinical practice.

The information contained in this book is intended only to inform and educate the
reader. It should not be considered as a substitute for the personal and private advice,
diagnosis, or treatment of a licensed physician or other health-care professional.

This book is printed on acid-free paper.

To my father, Alvin Luftman, M.D., physician extraordinaire,
who appreciated women as being beautiful, bright, and capable.
To my mother, Barbara, a role model of a loving, beautiful,
and brilliant woman.
To Harlan, Jessica, and Spencer—you are the beauty in my life.
—Debi

To Mark: Your enthusiasm and drive are contagious.
To Marissa: Your ability to see and create beauty in the world
is truly remarkable.
To Gigi: Kiss, hug, love. To my mother, Jean, and Aunt Mikki:
Two remarkable women and role models who broke through
the glass ceilings, allowing me and all women so many
more opportunities.
—Eva

CONTENTS

Acknowledgments   vii

Introduction: You're 20 Percent More
Beautiful than You Think   xi

PART 1

THE REAL LAW OF ATTRACTION

Chapter 1 Beauty: Skin Deep and Deeper   3

Chapter 2 The Beauty-Brain Loop   27

Chapter 3 The Beauty Prescription Quiz   47

PART 2

LIVING THE BEAUTY-BRAIN LOOP

Chapter 4 Inner Beauty: It All Begins Here   75

Chapter 5 Health: The Five Cards of Lifelong Wellness   97

Chapter 6 Outer Beauty: It's OK to Want to Look Fantastic   127

Chapter 7 Environment: Living in the World You Make   169

PART

3

BEAUTIFUL FOR LIFE

Chapter 8 Staying Beautiful Through the Years   191

Chapter 9 Beauty 911: Being Your Best During Times
of Transition   215

Chapter 10 Secrets to Lending Nature a Hand   241

Chapter 11 Wearing Pearls with Scrubs   265

Appendix: Shopping the Beauty Counter with Dr. Debra   275

Notes   285

Resources   291

Index   295

ACKNOWLEDGMENTS

OUR GRATITUDE COULD be a book of its own.

This project probably would never have come to be had we not taken respite together at the home of a beautiful and generous woman, Mary Ellen Trainor. It was there in Jamaica where our children frolicked through waterfalls and our husbands barbecued local fish that we conceptualized *The Beauty Prescription.*

I thank my office staff, the people who do the real work: Debby Perry, Linda Fiscina, Jennifer Fuglevand, and Jenalle Devine. Kerry Schlosser and Dr. Jasmine Yun, without your help and excellent patient care, I would not have had time to consider writing a book.

To Lisa Gregorisch-Dempsey and Patti Jacobs, my L.A. Beauty Buddies, thank you for all your love and support and great lunches full of quick wit. Thanks to Lia and Murray Markiles for your Sunday "feedback," and to Ellen Deutchman, who always gave me her take on antiaging treatments even before she started aging. Thanks to Ann Flower, my great helper and contact in the beauty world. To the beautiful HHS ladies and Patti Toll for being my Beauty Buddies.

I owe a debt to Dr. Mark Nestor. Not only is he Eva's husband, but the perfect sounding board on all things related to dermatology, lasers, and cosmetic surgery. His knowledge and expertise are inspirational.

Thanks to Cindy Hassel and Karen Smalley for bringing beauty into our lives. To Steven, who understood beauty even as a child. Thank you to my original UCLA dermatology beauty buddies: Monica Dahlem, M.D., and Lisa Airan, M.D. Thanks to Lenore Kakita, M.D., for helping pave the way for women dermatologists who followed her.

I have endless gratitude for the fabulous women role models in my life: my aunt Renee, whose beauty, intelligence, artistic talent, and ability to make people around her feel special are true gifts; my aunt Edith, a woman before her time, mother of four boys, attorney, psychotherapist, glamorous lady, and an inspiration; my late aunt Betty, who saw beauty in music and her family; and most of all to my mother, Barbara, thank you for everything . . . literally.

Most important, I thank my family: My husband, Harlan, an incredible doctor and the original author in the family, saving lives in the ER, keeping me laughing, and supporting my projects. My children, Jessica and Spencer, thank you for being such amazing people. I am so proud of you and know you appreciate the beauty around you.

—*Debra Luftman, M.D.*

The phrase "it takes a village" represents profound wisdom. I have so many people in my village without whom this book could never have come to be. First, to my husband, Mark, I deeply appreciate that you opened your world of dermatology and shared your vision of beauty and aesthetics. And to my family, my "Miami family": Elaine and Irv Billings; Sherry, Danielle, and Brittany Castellanos; and Lindsay Murdock; and to my extended family scattered across the country, a world of gratitude for your constant love and support.

To my friends and advisers, Brooke Alexander, Bernard Beitman, Lisa Bloch, Jennifer Charyk, Karin Esposito, Larry Harmon, Ellen Helman, Fred Karlton, Stephanie Layton, Christian Leuzzi, Sherri Lewis Thomas, Tom Mahle, Gina Marcus, Mary Mayotte, Debbie and Adrian Muller, Hart Porsche, Gonzolo Quesada, Linda Radford, Rae Sanchini, Starr Sariego, and Nancy Scheinman. I am so blessed to have all of you in my life.

To my chairmen, Julio Licinio; Larry Schachner; and my colleagues at the Miller School of Medicine and Mount Sinai Medical Center: Sara Bodner, Elizabeth Crocco, David and Susan Loewenstein, Ilan Melnick, and Ray Ownby. Thank you for seeing the beauty in combining dermatology and psychiatry.

To my friends in the dermatology and aesthetics industry who bravely welcomed a psychiatrist into the fold and have supported this project in countless ways: Humberto and Erika Antunes, Louis Firina, Diane Foster, Paul Sowyrda, and Charles and Daneen Stiefel, Dale Weiss.

To my home and office assistants, without whom nothing would be beautiful: Cecilia and Christy Abadie, Rosa Chavez, Viviana Luz Hernandez, and Glennys Morale. To all of you, I am deeply grateful. Thanks for making my life beautiful.

—*Eva Ritvo, M.D.*

And from us both:

As in every story there is a beginning, a middle, and an end. In our book there is Hilary Johnson; Wendy Walsh, Ph.D.; and Tim Vandehey. Without this brilliant group there would be no beauty in our prescription. Tim, our collaborator, must be the most patient man alive. To deal with two mommy M.D.s—multitasking, adding, subtracting, and over all trying to just get it "write"(pun intended)—he just made it happen. For that we are forever grateful.

Our Beauty Buddies and the accomplished ladies who shared Beauty Pearls with us deserve special thanks for sharing their professional advice and exquisite stories. We thank all our contributors to our Beauty Prescription for sharing their thoughts with us.

Thank you to our agents, Jillian Manus and Dena Fischer, for believing in our concept of beauty inside and out. They went to bat for us always remembering our message, "There is no beauty without the brain." A special thanks to Lisa Bloch, who brought us to Jillian.

Thank you to Ann Flower for her creativity. To Lisa Gregorisch-Dempsey for making a dream a reality. Thanks to Judith McCarthy, publisher par excellence, who understood from the beginning that this was a different kind of beauty book and brought our ideas to life. We admire her foresight and dedication. Special thanks to our project editor, Nancy Hall, and book designer, Michael Rohani. You made our work sing. Thanks also to the marketing team at McGraw-Hill.

Finally, we wish to thank our patients. We're humbled by the trust you place in us, and we're honored to care for you. Thank you for sharing your lives with us. You have expanded our vision. This book is for all of you.

You're 20 Percent More Beautiful than You Think

*People often say that "beauty is in the eye of the
beholder," and I say that the most liberating thing
about beauty is realizing that you are the beholder.
This empowers us to find beauty in places where others
have not dared to look, including inside ourselves.*

—Salma Hayek

WE'RE GOING TO tell you how to make yourself 20 percent more beautiful in just a few seconds. Impossible? Well, let's give it a try. First, look in the mirror. Then, while assessing your image, factor in the premise that other people see you as 20 percent better-looking than you see yourself. It's true.

Combining what we have noted in our clinical experience with information from psychological studies, we find that women view themselves as approximately 20 percent less attractive than others perceive them. Your brain is a tougher critic of your looks than Simon Cowell, of "American Idol," could ever be. But you can make your brain your greatest beauty ally. By giving yourself permission to look in the mirror in a more positive way, you'll see yourself looking better already.

Why do you think you judge yourself to be 20 percent less attractive than others find you? Because in the mirror, you're just your looks. Many people stand before the glass as though they're having a mug shot taken. There's none of the personality, fire, or swagger that they exhibit in the real world. Your reflection is simply not the whole you. Others also see your charisma, wit, kindness, empathy, intellect, talent—whatever makes you special. You're far more than the sum of your parts. That's what the world sees.

That, in a nutshell, is *The Beauty Prescription*. There are many definitions of beauty and many ways to be beautiful. You've always known this, but in a culture filled with overpowering images of one kind of female beauty, it's easy to forget, making you feel inadequate. Our mission in this book is to remind you that though you can't change your genetic makeup, many of the most compelling aspects of beauty are completely within your power to change, bringing you benefits that are both more rewarding and more enduring: greater confidence, stronger self-esteem, better health, more joy from life, and lasting beauty that shines for everyone to see.

BEAUTY MATTERS

Why care about beauty? Because it really does have its privileges. You can see it all around you. Beautiful people earn more money and hold greater positions of power. Research shows that physically attractive people get special treatment from employers, strangers, criminal courts, potential mates . . . and even their own mothers! Beauty sets off complex reward circuitry in our brains that compels us to want what we deem as beautiful. Simply put, we like to please those who are good-looking, and we allow ourselves to be easily persuaded by them. Some studies show that we even make more room on the street for attractive folks. In reality, beauty isn't just some shallow preoccupation. It matters to all levels of society. Caring about being the most attractive woman that you can be does not make you vain. It makes you smart!

We come by this reverence for beauty naturally. For our hunter-gatherer ancestors, recognizing beauty meant survival. Beautiful skin, hair, nails, and teeth indicated good health and youthfulness—and ultimately reproductive capability. Beauty meant health, which meant more potential for offspring, some of whom would survive to perpetuate the species. We are genetically programmed to be attracted to beauty as a way to assess genetic fitness. Our need for and preoccupation with beauty resides in our DNA.

Humans are also awed by confidence and assertiveness—qualities that good-looking people tend to possess. Studies have shown that physically attractive people are more self-confident, more socially at ease, and less likely to worry about the negative opinions of others. They feel more in control of their lives and tend to be more forceful. It's not a coincidence that many highly successful, wealthy men and women also tend to be good-looking. While this can seem to be some kind of ridiculous good fortune—looks, money, and power: how lucky can one person be?—it's more likely that the physical appearance of movers and shakers produces a self-assurance that helps them get where and what they want.

As you can see, what's on the inside is deeply connected to what's on the outside. The two are so firmly joined that it's hard to know which comes first. But in the end, which is more important? Does external beauty create self-confidence, or does self-confidence look beautiful? The answer is *both*. Inner beauty and outer beauty complement each other in a "Beauty-Brain Loop." Teaching you how to make the loop work for you is the heart of *The Beauty Prescription*.

Seeing Yourself as a Work of Art

In this book, we approach beauty from a fresh direction, dividing it into two types: *innate beauty*, the physical beauty we're biologically configured to respond to, and *evolving beauty*, that which we find beautiful that changes over time as we mature and have different experiences.

How do you judge beauty in yourself, in others, and in the world? To find out, let's try a good, old-fashioned "bird-watching" exercise. Sit on a park bench for an hour in a busy area and watch each woman who walks by. Who do you rate as beautiful, and who do you rate as unattractive? Is your judgment based only on the figure, clothing, or face? Probably. Repeat the exercise, but this time, try to look for other qualities that define the women's attractiveness. Does a physically pretty woman have an ugly frown as she talks into her cell phone? Perhaps you'd rate her as unattractive. Maybe a young mother who's overweight shines with love and pleasure as she carries her laughing toddler. By a different standard, she's become beautiful. See what we're getting at? When you learn to judge beauty by standards beyond superficial physical appearance, more people—and more things—become beautiful. That's evolving beauty. Your perceptions of what's beautiful about you and others change as you change.

Once you find out where your knee-jerk "standards" are, you can begin to let them go. The best way to have more beauty in your life is to train yourself to see more of it. Imagine you are photographer Annie Leibovitz, looking for beauty, humanity, vulnerability, and tenderness in the parade that passes by. Hair-styles and five extra pounds start to seem irrelevant. Just as you start to see beauty in others, maybe you'll start to see yourself as less of a "weight" or a "blemish" and more of a work of art . . . in progress, of course.

As the years pass, our outer beauty frays around the edges. That's nothing to be ashamed of. In fact, it's all the more reason to take marvelous care of your body starting now, even if you're young. It's time we celebrate the lasting, soul-deep gorgeousness that comes with knowing yourself, loving who you've become, and inhabiting your skin with grace, élan, and sex appeal—no matter how old you are. Although the primal reproductive urge may make sex hot and lusty when you're twenty-two, sex is often best later in life as we come to know ourselves and our partners better.

If you're twenty-five, aging skin may not even be on your radar screen, so you may think this book is not for you. Think again. In an interconnected world, we're all competing more intensely than ever for jobs and mates. In that competition, beauty is cur-rency. Still, that's not the main reason to care about looking and being your best. All women of substance, whether they're twenty or sixty-five, want to be cherished for their inner radiance as well as their appearance. Even very attractive women don't want to be seen as just pretty faces. We've all fought hard for our educations, career achievements, laugh lines, and spiritual revelations. We all crave recognition of the kind of beauty that reveals itself in the body, mind, and spirit of a woman who is at peace with her age, her health, her relationships, and her path.

How This Book Came to Be

Over twenty-five years, Debra, a board-certified dermatologist with a background in internal medicine, and Eva, a board-certified psychiatrist, carried on a dialogue that would become *The Beauty Prescription*. While on a beach vacation (under an umbrella and wearing SPF 45 sunscreen, naturally), we came to realize that even though we had different specialties, we were treating the same patients with many of the same concerns. In this way, we saw the powerful correlation between self-esteem (Eva's patients' concern) and physical appearance (Debra's patients' concern). When we added our own life experiences to the mix, we recognized a wonderful synergy between our two specialties.

From our perspective, there's a profound physical connection between the brain and beauty. The same fetal tissue that formed your brain and nervous system also formed your skin. Endorphins, those happy endogenous opioid hormones made by the brain, spark a sense of euphoria while making your skin glow. Stress not only sends your brain into agitation but also pumps up the body's production of cortisol, a hormone that thins the skin and increases the activity of the sebaceous glands, causing acne and rosacea. Brain foods such as omega-3-rich salmon, green tea, and water are beneficial for your skin. Your mind and appearance are intertwined in ways that science is only beginning to understand.

So, we started asking questions about beauty: What is it? Who defines it? How does it pressure women? How does it free women? How does it empower women? How is beauty related to health? Why do some less attractive women feel so great about their looks while some beautiful women feel so unattractive? How can every woman attain a better balance?

We noticed that as our patients received help in one area, they improved in the other. Women who did the cognitive work to cope with their anxieties in a healthy manner also took better care of themselves and became more attractive. Others who lost weight or received long-overdue skin care developed stronger self-esteem. It became clear to us that in beauty, the physical and mental are inextricably linked. When you feel more beautiful, you *are* more beautiful. That is the Beauty-Brain Loop in action.

BEAUTY BUDDIES

Of course, we're not just the authors of this book. We've lived it. We've been best friends since medical school and stayed that way through marriages, kids, teaching, and practices, one in Beverly Hills and the other in Miami—what we call the Botox Latitudes. We've watched each other age and put in more time, effort, and money to be able to look the way we want to look. We've listened to each other lament pregnancy pounds that were slow to come off and skin that isn't as smooth as when we met.

At the same time, we've watched each other become dedicated physicians. We've raised families, given back to our communities, and grown in kindness, judgment, and self-confidence. We're constantly in the process of becoming the women we want to be, despite endless hours of multitasking between career demands and family. With the years has come wisdom about maximizing our beauty strengths and minimizing our weaknesses. We know our strong points, and we know when our inner critic is taking cheap shots, so we can tune her out.

We're living the principles of *The Beauty Prescription*. One way we have coped with life's ups and downs is by maintaining our close friendship. We call ourselves "beauty buddies." We've found that lots of women are "beauty buddies"—longtime friends who share beauty regimens and support each other as they work toward their inner and outer goals. In the coming chapters, you'll meet a wide range of beauty buddies, some of them famous, others people we know—best friends, mothers and daughters. You'll read about how they're there for each other at the gym or the hair salon, and in times when they might not be at their most beautiful. We think you'll find them as inspiring as we do.

Having beauty buddies isn't just about being social. Being with other women actually makes us feel better. A UCLA study conducted in 2002 suggests that friendships between women release more of the hormone oxytocin, which counters stress hormones and promotes relaxation. So, that wonderful belonging, loved feeling you get from going to the spa with your best friend isn't all in your head. It's caused by chemicals sent throughout your body that support your mental and physical health and make you look better in the process.

In addition to beauty buddies, we have included some beauty secrets throughout the book to help you on your journey:

- **Beauty Stories:** Real-life clinical examples, composites of some of our own patients whose problems and resolutions offer lessons about becoming more beautiful inside and out.

- **Beauty Boosters:** Practical, low-cost "quick fixes" you can use to make yourself look and feel better fast, such as getting a massage to help you relax and switching to a whitening toothpaste. From simple dietary changes to fast mood enhancers, you'll glean plenty of helpful ideas.
- **Beauty Busters:** Myths about beauty, mental health, and cosmetic medicine abound. Some of them are silly, while others are harmful or downright dangerous. We'll debunk them all in these informative sidebars.
- **Beauty Pearls:** Throughout the book, we've scattered sidebars from prominent women—celebrities, beauty insiders, beauty editors. They share their views on what makes a woman beautiful.
- **Beauty and the Brain Rx:** Specific steps you can take to move toward a more beautiful you, inside and out.
- **Beauty Bullets:** A quick summary of the major points of each chapter.

It's OK to Want to Look Great

Our goal for this book is nothing less than to redefine what it means to be beautiful. We hope you'll reach the last page with some handy tools to help you gain a strong balance of inner and outer beauty. It's OK to care about looking great . . . as long as that's not all you care about. Your physical appearance speaks volumes about you—your habits, diet, exercise, emotional state, how happy you are in your job and relationships, what you think of yourself as you lie in your bed at night, and more. How you think and feel affects how you look. So, as you work on your inner being, remember that your outer being will transform for the better. That's good news. It means that all of us can charm the socks off everyone if we're aglow with radiant health and inner peace.

We want you to become the woman that actress Claudette Colbert had in mind when she said, "It matters more what's in a woman's face than what's on it." That's accessible to every one of us. Let's get started.

part 1

The Real
Law of
Attraction

1

Beauty: Skin Deep and Deeper

Nothing makes a woman more beautiful than the belief that she is beautiful.

—Sophia Loren

THE TWO OF us have been linked all our lives by some amazing synchronicities. We grew up less than ten miles from each other and both went to high schools in "the Valley" in Los Angeles, only five miles apart. This was the era of malls, big hair, and the song "Valley Girl." Debra grew up in Laurel Canyon, in the Hollywood hills, when Carole King and Joni Mitchell lived there; Eva grew up in Encino, where the movie *Fast Times at Ridgemont High* was set and Valleyspeak originated ("whatever"). We didn't know each other until we were both in Boston for medical school, but we definitely orbited each other's worlds.

More coincidences? Both sets of parents are in medicine. Eva's parents are both psychiatrists. Debra's dad was an ob-gyn, and her mother is a registered nurse with a master's degree in public health. Talk about the apple not falling far from the tree! But it gets better. Today, Debra's husband is an ER physician. Eva's husband? A dermatologist. More often than not, we show up places wearing almost identical outfits. At first, we couldn't figure out who was copying whom, but now that we are separated by three thousand miles, we realize that these coincidences are just part of our special connection.

The point is that we've been close for a long time. We've always been there to support each other during good times and bad. We work hard to make each other feel beautiful inside and out. When one of us is down on herself, the other has always come through with a kind word, a beauty break, or a bit of wisdom, all of which put things in perspective.

We want to help other women the way we have helped each other. For inspiration, take a look at the Sophia Loren quote again. It's easy for one of the world's great beauties to say, but she's right. When you feel wonderful about yourself, you radiate beauty, even if you're jogging to the corner Starbucks on Sunday morning in your sweats, your unwashed hair pulled back with one of those clips you use to keep bags of potato chips closed.

Now multiply that idea by about six billion, and you get the full scope of what we consider to be truly beautiful about the world's most amazing women (and men): because they love themselves, they can lavish affection on all the people around them as well. Kindness, compassion, positive energy—these are the hallmarks of lasting beauty that goes far beyond the temporary virtues of a toned body and flawless skin.

THE BEAUTY REGIMEN EVERY WOMAN CAN AFFORD

Every time you fly, a flight attendant reminds you that should those yellow oxygen masks drop from the ceiling, you're to get your own mask on before you help your child or ailing grandmother. Sounds callous, but it's smart advice. You can't help anyone else until you take care of yourself. Women who abuse their bodies and are under too much stress end up neglecting themselves, and it's a short step from there to neglecting others. When you're hypercritical every time you step in front of a mirror, it's hard to love yourself, never mind being a good spouse, boss, or coworker. It becomes easy to let yourself and your relationships slide.

Mind you, we're certainly not against using the science of beauty to look your best. Cosmetic procedures and modern medicine can play a major role in helping you look great, provided you use them as part of a physically and mentally healthful program of self-care. But given how expensive cosmetic medicine and personal trainers can be, many women become discouraged and think they can't be more attractive. That's a mistake, because the most effective beauty regimen in the world doesn't cost a dime and is available to any woman, anywhere: unstoppable, radiant self-esteem.

If that's the case, then why are women still obsessed with big breasts, flat stomachs, and perfect noses? Why haven't self-confident, passionate women of every size and shape replaced bikini-clad, size-two twenty-year-olds on our magazine covers? Are women just shallow? Not at all. It's a response to millions of years of evolutionary programming that's embedded a craving for beauty into human DNA. So, if you feel bad because the young, gorgeous girl in the minidress is getting all the stares, do what we do. Blame Darwin. Then move on.

FITTING INTO OUR GENES

In her book *Survival of the Prettiest,* Dr. Nancy Etcoff gets right to the point: "Beauty is a universal part of human experience . . . it provokes pleasure, rivets attention, and impels actions that help ensure the survival of our genes. Our extreme sensitivity to beauty is hardwired, that is, governed by circuits in the brain shaped by natural selection. We love to look at smooth skin, thick shiny hair, curved waists, and symmetrical bodies because in the course of evolution the people who noticed these signals and desired their possessors had more reproductive success."

In other words, beauty has a genetic purpose: to send signals to potential mates that one is healthy and able to bear and raise healthy children to carry on the mate's DNA. That's why men have always found women in their late teens and early twenties alluring: that's the age when their faces and bodies are most loudly broadcasting the signals that they are vital and fertile and will be so long enough to successfully raise the babies to young adulthood. People aren't always aware of the reasons behind their feelings of attraction, of course. Certainly, no man looks at a stunning young woman and thinks, "Wow, she will be a great vessel for my genetic material," but that is what our genes know.

Ever wonder why older-man/younger-woman pairings are so common, from the "trophy wife" trend to Hollywood hookups? It's the mating instinct. Women are unique among mammals in that their fertility peaks early and declines fairly rapidly. Men maintain their fertility throughout their lives; thus, age does not factor in as much when women seek male partners. Women tend to look for other qualities that indicate a man has the ability to protect and provide for them and their offspring: size, vitality, prosperity, and stability. Thus, mating with a fifty-five-year-old man who has wealth and status might make perfect sense to a thirty-year-old woman who still has her luminous looks.

Also, our programming to prefer "averageness" makes the familiar look good to us. Standards change over time as certain

BEAUTY BUDDIES

Lisa Gregorisch-Dempsey, senior executive producer, EXTRA TV;
Patti Jacobs, M.D., mother of four and an internist

Both busy women in demanding fields, Lisa and Patti met through a family connection (Lisa is Patti's husband's cousin) and bonded quickly over coffee. "Lisa is my Beauty Buddy because she is beautiful!" says Patti. "We started off meeting at the corner coffee shop, catching up about family and getting to know each other. One on one was totally different from when the whole family got together."

"Yeah, we could never get a word in edgewise around the rest of the family," says Lisa. "From coffees, we graduated to lunches, so they would last longer. We had so much more in common than we imagined we had. I don't have kids; Patti has four. I have a fast-paced career in entertainment; Patti is a doctor who stopped working to raise her kids."

One day, the two women realized they were talking about much more than simple beauty tips—they were exchanging ideas on how to make life more beautiful.

"We used to smile politely across the room at family functions," says Lisa, "and now we check out each other's smile lines. But at our lunches, how is it that we always seem to wind up at the brightest lunch spot in town, and I always get the window seat? I am the oldest, and sunlight is not my friend!"

"Oh stop," says Patti. "I can barely remember where we go or what we eat. I just love the time we spend unwinding and catching up. One thing other women can learn from us is that sometimes we enjoy most the people we start out knowing the least."

characteristics become the norm, such as straight white teeth, wrinkle-free skin, and large breasts. The more people who possess these characteristics, the more attractive they become.

WHY A BEAUTIFUL WOMAN IS LIKE A LOTTERY WIN

This genetic preoccupation with beauty goes back as far as recorded history. Red ochre paints more than forty thousand years old have been discovered in southern Africa, leading anthropologists to surmise that they were used for facial or body ornamentation. There is evidence that men and women in fourth-century Nubia tattooed their bodies.

The Roman author Ovid wrote the first book on cosmetics, *The Art of Beauty*, in 5 B.C., detailing the use of black eye shadow made from wood ash and golden eye shadow made from saffron. Two-thousand-year-old face creams, cosmetic boxes, and shaving sets have been unearthed in archaeological sites in Egypt, some believed to belong to the legendary Queen Nefertiti. You get the picture. We've been trying to enhance our appearance—and attract the attention of possible mates—for a long, long time, and this drive is unlikely to go away soon.

Fast-forward to today, and we haven't come a long way, baby. According to analysts at Goldman Sachs, worldwide spending on beauty products has rocketed to more than $95 billion a year— $24 billion for skin-care products, $18 billion for makeup, $38 billion for hair-care products, and $15 billion for fragrance. In the United States, we spend more on beauty products than on social services and education *combined*. According to *The Economist* (we just love this), Brazil now has nine hundred thousand Avon ladies—more people than it has in its army and navy combined. The global beauty market is growing at 7 percent per year, more than the GDP growth rate of the world's developing nations.

We spend and fret so much for a simple reason: beauty gets rewarded. In a 2001 study at Massachusetts General Hospital and Harvard Medical School, when young men viewed images of attractive female faces, functional magnetic resonance imaging (MRI) showed that the brain's "reward circuitry" lit up like a Christmas tree. The men's brains released a cascade of dopamine, the same pleasure hormone released when we have sex, eat delicious food, take cocaine, or make money. So, when a man tells you your beauty is intoxicating, it's not just a cheesy line—well, it might be; that's another book—but an honest assessment of the effect you're having on his brain.

THE BEAUTIFUL PEOPLE REALLY ARE DIFFERENT

Ready for some righteous outrage? Good-looking men and women in our society are rewarded just for being beautiful. Study after study affirms that attractive people are treated better than their average-looking peers. Beautiful people hold higher positions of power, get special treatment from employers and total strangers, and even enjoy greater leniency from criminal courts! A 2007 study by researchers at the University of California revealed that the most attractive people in the workplace earn 12 percent more than those who are average in appearance. Moreover, beautiful folks score higher on exams and are more likely to get away with shoplifting.

Psychologist Judith Langlois performed an experiment in which she showed hundreds of photos of adult faces to babies from three to six months old. The babies stared longer at the faces that adults rated as attractive. Likewise, one-year-old babies have been shown to play longer with attractive dolls. Evolutionary psychologist Satoshi Kanazawa, of the London School of Economics, even found that attractive women are more likely to give birth to attractive daughters, who in turn become more likely to have beautiful offspring, and so on and so on. Similar studies have shown that tall men with high social status have more male offspring. The "pretty gene" is being passed on in women, and the "provider gene" is being passed down in men, so that with each new generation, the chances of success increase. Ever wondered why the people in old paintings are so much less attractive and shorter than our contemporaries? That's evolution at work.

There's even a growing body of evidence suggesting that attractive people tend to live better and longer. In one study,

---

 ## BEAUTY BOOSTERS

Practical things you can do now to be more beautiful

Stop the negative, self-critical obsessing about yourself. That will show on your face in the form of frown lines and other expressions you may not even be aware of. Instead, focus on others. With every interaction, think about ways to make the other person feel wanted and liked. When you catch yourself wondering if someone is noticing your flaws, immediately look for something positive about the person, and verbalize the compliment. In this way, thoughts such as "Does she see my pimples?" can become "I like your new hairstyle!" or "Great jacket!" This takes the pressure off you and rewires your brain to think positively. Positive thinking is attractive!

twenty undergraduates rated fifty high school yearbook photos from the 1920s for attractiveness. The people who were rated as more attractive had indeed lived longer, and the male raters' assessment of attractiveness was correlated even more with longevity. Another study looked at one thousand men and found that those who appeared older than their chronological age actually *were* older according to key physiological markers. The genetically blessed members of society have also been found to be less lonely, less socially nervous, more popular, more socially skilled, and more sexually experienced than the less fortunate populace. Good looks, brains, and success do often go together.

INNATE BEAUTY

It may be easy to conclude from all these studies and surveys that humans are self-deluded, pheromone-sniffing apes enslaved to a cruel ancestral heritage. Cheer up. That's part of the story, but not the whole story. We're sharing the Darwinian foundation of beauty with you to emphasize that beauty really does matter—and that improving your inner and outer beauty can have a positive effect on the quality of your life. The rest of the story features a deeper, more personal aspect to beauty that has everything to do with the natural human tendency to strive for what's higher and nobler in us all.

There are two ways of recognizing beauty in ourselves and in others. *Innate beauty*, which elicits the hardwired biological response just discussed, is the more obvious of the two. People are preconditioned, even at birth, to enjoy the sight of a specific set of physical characteristics. We carry a prototype of what is attractive in our DNA. It's why certain people who fit our biological ideal of beauty can have such a powerful effect on us, and it's also what makes us look in the mirror and criticize ourselves when we don't fit that archetype.

In a massive study of thirty-seven cultures from tribal to modern, researchers found that all men prefer the same things: full lips; clear, healthy skin; lustrous hair; good muscle tone; youthful gait; animated facial expression; and a high energy level.

✒ BEAUTY STORY: "KAREN"

Karen had been married to a professional man for more than twenty-five years. She gave up her professional life to become a full-time wife and mother. Not long after their daughter left for college, her husband came home one day and dropped this bomb: "Our marriage is over. I want to move on." He was having an affair with a younger woman. The news was devastating.

Karen realized that in working for so many years to take care of her family, she had let herself go physically. She felt that this was why her husband had left her—he didn't find her physically attractive anymore, and their sex life had been practically nonexistent. She came to see Debra wanting, she said, to "fix myself up," which can often be code for "give me emergency cosmetic surgery that will make me look and feel better about myself immediately!" Instead, Karen agreed that she would do some work on her emotional state and her self-esteem, and then she and Debra would discuss cosmetic improvements.

Karen spent the next six months working with a therapist to address her anger, humiliation, and poor self-esteem. Following her therapy, with a better personal equilibrium, she came back to Debra and had some cosmetic work done.

Debra: *It is common for patients to want to deal with years of neglect in a single visit. I'm always skeptical when patients who have never had any cosmetic work show up and want an immediate makeover. I try to understand their motivation. You have to look at the cause of the problem and help them with that.*

Eva: *Sometimes, it takes a crisis for people to want to make changes. Other times, people run up against what I call "life markers." Women are coming up to some milestone—a high school reunion, turning forty, an anniversary, a child's bar mitzvah—and they know that they've neglected themselves for a long time. They suddenly say, "I've got to do something about this now!"*

For men, innate beauty is highly visual. Ad agencies take advantage of this in advertising for shiny luxury cars, plasma TVs, and the like. Men are also innately programmed to respond to variety. Women trying to attract a man will get new hairstyles, wear different jewelry, update their wardrobes—anything to stimulate that reward circuitry that's keyed to variety. Men have a minimal investment in creating new offspring (after all, they can plant their seed and move on), so for them it pays to explore many options.

EVOLVING BEAUTY

We aren't completely under the sway of our biology, however. If we were, every man over fifty would dump his wife the minute she hit menopause and run off with some young gal. That happens, but far more often, couples grow old together despite whatever evolutionary urges may pop up. Another aspect of beauty is at work here.

That's *evolving beauty*. Evolving beauty is our beauty software, and as with computer software, it's reprogrammable. This type of beauty is all about the aspects of the brain that change as we mature, become more self-aware, and have more life experiences. As you expand your ideas about what you consider beautiful, you perceive more beauty in yourself and in the world around you. You become like an art aficionado who has the opportunity to collect and appreciate more compositions with each passing year.

Most important, evolving beauty is about learning to perceive yourself holistically and appreciate many aspects of yourself as beautiful, not just your face and body. As we develop greater confidence, worldliness, wit, passion, style, and caring for others, we see those qualities as making us more attractive and desirable. Because we feel more beautiful, other people perceive us in the same way. We don't all look like high-fashion models, yet most of us acquire a mate and have children. Women all over the world of every shape and size find wonderful partners who think they are gorgeous.

"Susan" is an example of this. She is the kind of woman we've all known at one time or another. She is not beautiful in the fashion-magazine sense. She's carrying too much weight, she doesn't have a hairstyle, and her wardrobe would make a thrift store owner go pale. Nevertheless, at any social gathering, she's the center of attention. Men flock to her; people can't take their eyes off her. She's *sexy*. Why? Because she's completely at home in her skin. She loves herself, and that love radiates to everyone around her. She's funny and bawdy and sweet. She has *made* herself into an attractive woman by the force of her personality, confidence, and charm. Susan has a highly evolved appreciation of beauty in herself and in those around her. Her outgoing personality and confidence resonate with men and women, because they have learned that being around women like Susan is pleasurable.

Evolving beauty comes to the forefront as you age and mature. Purely physical beauty holds sway in your youth, because those are your reproductive years, but physical beauty peaks in your twenties, so as you get older, evolving beauty takes center stage. As the years pass, you learn to take better care of yourself. You can't just throw on a pair of jeans and a T-shirt, leave the house without makeup, and look stunning. You need a winning personality and a ready sense of humor to accessorize your looks. Evolving beauty peaks when a woman loves who she is and feels confident about the choices she has made—when she's radiantly happy with her life and leaves the house knowing she looks her best, can engage others with a dynamic laugh and a captivating story, and has a style all her own.

THE *REAL* LAW OF ATTRACTION

In this light, it's necessary to understand the differences among *beauty*, *attractiveness*, and *magnetism*. Innate beauty is the most basic level, the stuff of biology and fertility. You can do much to make yourself more beautiful—from working out and getting in shape, to having your makeup professionally applied, to undergoing cosmetic surgery—but the genetic hand you're dealt still governs.

Attractiveness is another matter. Here, the sky is the limit. You become attractive when you combine looking your best with a joyful sense of self-love and peace with who you are and where you are in your life.

Then comes magnetism. This is the state we hope *The Beauty Prescription* will help you reach. A magnetic woman takes attractiveness and adds a burst of energy directed at those around her. She's charismatic and self-assured. She loves everybody and makes people feel better about themselves. She has presence. Like a magnet, she *attracts* people wherever she goes. That's the true "law of attraction." Magnetism is evolving beauty that becomes richer and more radiant as you become healthier, more self-aware, and more passionate about life.

A perfect example is Elaine Billings, who, at seventy, works in a Florida dermatologist's office and takes exceptional pride in her appearance. "At my age, it's that much more important for me to look great," she says. "But first you have to have a secure feeling about yourself and other people. You go forward from there. I want to look good. I have more energy than people in this office who are twenty-five."

Magnetism is the quality that blends being perfectly put together with total self-confidence and pure, unadulterated charm. Think fashion doyenne Coco Chanel. The French have a term for women of her type: *jolie laide*. It means, literally, "beautiful ugly." Coco Chanel, who may well be the most stylish woman ever to have lived, didn't have the voluptuous figure or soft features favored in her era. She was thin and bony, with pinched facial features, but she was always the most vivid and interesting creature in the room, with a bold, eccentric style all her own. She was magnetic.

In one revealing study, psychologists videotaped people as they entered a room and introduced themselves. They then asked strangers to watch the video and rate the people on physical attractiveness, emotional expressiveness, and social skills. In determining likability, physical appearance was the *least* important factor. Charm trumps beauty every time.

GIVING YOURSELF A "FAITH LIFT"

You know Faith Hill. Country music superstar, great beauty—like Mary Poppins, "practically perfect in every way." You may recall when a story broke on network television that a cover photo of her on a major women's magazine had been heavily doctored. It's common knowledge that magazines digitally retouch photos, even when the images are of people who are exceptionally attractive. In this case, the Photoshop expert cleared her skin of wrinkles and pores, thinned her arms, and made her face appear slimmer. The overall effect was to make an already beautiful woman into a "perfect beauty." The editors were trying to appeal to our hardwired ideal of beauty. Natural beauty wasn't good enough for their readers. They demanded perfection.

What surprised the two of us was the uproar over the retouching. It made the "Today Show." The impression was that people all over the country were shocked—shocked!—that a magazine cover had been doctored. As if anyone believes that the men and women who stare back at us from the supermarket checkout lines actually look that way when they roll out of bed in the morning. But apparently, that's what many people must have been thinking.

OK, so somewhere deep down we know that perfect beauty is an illusive quality and that no one can really look like a perfect ten. Despite that knowledge, our sense of innate beauty still responds to the ideal of physical attractiveness. We can't help but look at the beautiful people. The media feed our desire to see ideal beauty. We all have the same beauty ideal in mind, which is why Barbie hasn't changed in forty years.

Even though we know that gorgeous celebrities are aided by makeup experts, professional lighting, costumers, cosmetic surgery, crash diets, and skilled photographers, we ache to look the way they do. We fixate on beautiful people, so magazine art directors feel pressured to make the naturally gorgeous Faith Hill artificially perfect; natural doesn't cut it. We're drawn to a standard of beauty that we know is as genuine as a three-dollar bill, yet we can't seem to help wanting to do almost anything to look that good. Our "gatherer" gene may have evolved into a "shopping" gene, but women still have a biological imperative to be attractive to potential mates.

For every woman like Diane Keaton, who's sexy and proud and who looked incredible in a daring nude scene in the movie *Something's Gotta Give*, hundreds are obsessed with getting their "flaws" erased. Our goal in this book is to help restore some of the faith all women should have in their own ability to feel and look their best, their way.

You're probably doing a lot of things right already, things that help you look great and feel wonderful about yourself. It's our job to help you understand these strengths before we take a look at where you can improve. It's time you realized that you can be magnificent on your own terms. It's about time you got a "faith lift."

PULLING YOURSELF UP BY YOUR OWN BRA STRAPS

A faith lift has nothing to do with religion or surgery. It's about believing in your ability to do things that make you as beautiful as you can be. Start with what you're doing right now. You're reading this book.

Think of it as pulling yourself up by your bra straps. That takes faith—faith in who you are and who you can become, faith in your ability to change things that may seem impossible, and faith in the idea that other people can see you differently from how they do today. So, before we move along, brava to you for taking this big step.

The real courage, however, comes when you develop the self-awareness to admit where you need help in your life. Whether the issue is psychological, such as low self-esteem or relationship problems, or dermatological, such as sun-damaged skin or aging, many women we treat do not realize that their actions and attitudes are causing their troubles. The solution may not be a pill or

---

BEAUTY BUSTERS

Beauty myths debunked while you wait

Myth: Small, gradual changes are always easier to make and sustain.
Fact: Often, it's easier to make big, bold changes all at once rather than ease into change in moderation. Making bold changes all at once, such as joining a gym and enrolling in a challenging aerobics class right away, yields instant positive feedback, both internal and external, which helps provide the motivation to continue the process of change. You feel that you're actually making some progress, perhaps in more than one area. When you make change more radical, you also create a stronger sense of investment in what you're doing, so it becomes harder to quit. Positive feedback from others around you can also help to sustain your motivation. Dieting and exercising together are far more effective than either alone.

a peel, but a commonsense suggestion to exercise and eat better, wear sunscreen, or work on changing defeatist patterns of thinking. Sometimes, that's not what people want to hear, but often, the best medicine we can deliver is a dose of reality: *if you want things to change, it starts with you.*

PUTTING HER BEST FACE FORWARD

Valerie Walker, director of the UCLA Medical Alumni Association, was diagnosed in 2001 with rosacea, a skin disease that causes acnelike breakouts and redness. Rosacea can have serious social and psychological consequences as sufferers become self-conscious about their appearance, especially when they are under stress, which makes outbreaks worse. The fact that people often associate the classic rosacea red nose (think W. C. Fields) with alcoholism doesn't help.

When Valerie was diagnosed, she was going through a personal crisis. She explains, "Coping with rosacea only exacerbated my stress level and undermined my self-esteem." She stopped looking in mirrors for fear that her face would be red and didn't want to have her photo taken, because it would be a reminder. "For years, I was too embarrassed to tell people I had rosacea," she says. "Little did I know that keeping it a secret only increased the symptoms. I found myself flushing badly in stressful situations. It affected my professional and personal lives. Then I thought, 'Having rosacea is not a reflection of the person I am. I *have* the disease; I am not the disease.'" Valerie decided to share her secret with a close friend, who confided that she, too, had rosacea. This was the turning point.

From that moment on, Valerie made the decision not to let rosacea affect her life and self-image in a negative way. She

---

BEAUTY PEARLS

What makes a woman beautiful? I think it's her presence rather than her physical characteristics. It's the presence of grace and poise and a kind of feminine strength. I find beauty in the fully rounded character of the feminine. Appreciating beauty on the campaign trail is what keeps me going. When I stand in front of people I appreciate it; I see the beauty in each person, in the heart of the people. I acknowledge the grace that's in each person in the room. His or her potential could be seen as beauty empowered, but it's greatly beyond the physical. It goes into the heart and the integrity of the individual.

Beauty is often associated with women, and I only associated it with women until I met my husband. He embodies those characteristics that could only be called beautiful.

—Elizabeth Kucinich,
wife of Congressman Dennis Kucinich (D-Ohio)

---

reports, "As I slowly 'let out the dancing ghosts,' I noticed I wasn't flushing as much. If I did, people knew why I was getting red and didn't comment about it." She has also learned to put her disease in perspective. "I've changed my inner monologue and am eager to discover ways to feel good about myself," she says. "A friend taught me how to put makeup on well, so the foundation cancels out the red. I call it putting my best face forward."

Six years after Valerie was diagnosed, she was asked to tape an infomercial for the skin-care product line Eucerin. This was a moment of truth. By saying yes, she banished the remaining ghosts, and the disease no longer has control over her life.

WHAT ARE YOU DOING RIGHT?

Valerie's change in mind produced changes in her body and her environment. Balanced beauty can be achieved by using the Beauty-Brain Loop. We will explain the loop in the next chapter. Its four stages revolve around your ability to do the following:

- Look at yourself honestly and see where you need to make changes
- Take positive steps to bring out your greatest inner and outer beauty
- Impact your health and environment in a positive way
- Maintain those changes for your whole life

The Beauty Prescription is about celebrating all the steps you're taking today, possibly without even knowing how good they are, to make yourself as beautiful as you can be. You're going to add to your life, not just subtract. A faith lift is confronting your feelings about yourself and trusting that you do have the power to make yourself a better woman—with you and no one else defining what "better" means.

THINGS ARE CHANGING

The good news is that the rapidly shifting landscape—including new scientific and medical research—gives women more ways than ever to be healthier and to look and feel better than at any time in the past. The bad news? Well, it's the same. The flow of new information and opportunity is a little dizzying. Some of the medical data are contradictory, and many of the new products and "miracle cures" are merely marketing gimmicks rather than substantial tools for self-improvement.

Today's women know better, and technology has provided us with more and better options. We understand how vital it is to care for our bodies and minds all our lives. Medical science has helped us learn about the foods that contribute to increased health and vitality. We have an array of vitamins and natural supplements at our fingertips. Complementary medicine such as acupuncture not only is more available but also is backed by mainstream research. We exercise like athletes without worrying that we'll become muscle-bound and less feminine. We're wiser than ever about the importance of sleep, relaxation, and finding joy and peace in our lives. Women are healthier, more beautiful, and more empowered than ever before in history. You are part of that wave of change.

You Are More Beautiful Today

We're still evolving. Living in a globalized world where there's so much visual stimulus, we're becoming more visual. Our brains are actually changing. We're becoming more attuned to how we can look our best and accentuate our best features. We're swimming in information from books, the media, the Internet, and beyond, and as a result, we're getting more educated and taking interest in new things throughout life, keeping our brains stimulated and healthy.

Women have more medical options, not just for cosmetic surgery but also for nonsurgical procedures and professional-quality beauty products that rejuvenate the skin instead of just hiding damage. These options gives today's woman the ability to eat better, get and stay in shape, and remain vibrant longer than her grandmother would have dreamed. Even cosmetics and fashions are evolving, thanks to an emphasis on natural ingredients and the influence of global culture. Right now, right here, you have everything you need not just to look your best but also to *be your best.*

Perhaps most important, though, is the recognition in our society that we need a holistic ideal of beauty instead of a harsh, punitive one that leads to eating disorders and excessive surgeries. We think it's time for a standard that recognizes the beauty of what's inside a woman as well as what's on the outside, and how they are forever intertwined.

Afghan rugs are justifiably famous for their quality and beauty, but they all have a tiny secret. Each weaver places one small flaw in the weave, as a symbol of the belief that humans cannot create perfection. It is for these flaws that these works of art are celebrated. We should be the same way, celebrating ourselves for the imperfections that make us unique. As the British psychologist and author Havelock Ellis said, "The absence of flaw in beauty is itself a flaw." Here's to the unique, splendid beauty in each one of us.

Beauty Bullets

ॐ Beauty has a biological purpose: reproduction.

ॐ Being beautiful really does make life better.

ॐ How you feel and who you are determine how other people see you more than your physical appearance.

- There are two kinds of beauty: innate, inborn sense of beauty, and evolving beauty that changes over time as you change.

- Being attractive and magnetic is more important than simple physical beauty—charm trumps beauty.

- We tend to delude ourselves that artificially created images of beauty are what we should aspire to.

- The "faith lift" is about having faith in yourself and your ability to make changes and become beautiful inside and out.

- Self-awareness is the key to change.

- You're probably already doing a lot of good things that you don't even realize are beneficial.

 ## BEAUTY AND THE BRAIN Rx

Empowerment

Dr. Eva: *Consider the messages about beauty and physical attractiveness that you received from your family and culture growing up. Did adults put down attractive girls as being superficial or not smart enough? Or, were looks emphasized too much in your household? Write down five thoughts about your appearance. Now write down five thoughts about your inner self (personality, feelings, and behaviors). Are these thoughts too negative?*

(continued)

Too positive? We are usually too critical. Now rework your ten comments, trying to be as accurate as possible. Don't be afraid to list your best features inside and out that contribute to your attractiveness. It's important to expand on the positives as we try to improve on our negative areas.

Dr. Debra: *Look in the mirror. List five positive physical features, and then list two features you'd like to improve. Ask yourself if these enhancements are realistic and if your choice is based on your own wishes, not the desire to please someone else. Finally, begin to train your eye to see a richer definition of beauty. Why do artists see more beauty in the world than other people? Answer: they look for it. The first step toward beauty is to teach yourself to see more beauty in the world around you. Take up painting, gardening, design, or even cake decorating. Learn to appreciate shape, color, and texture. All of this trains your eye beyond the one-note beauty of the fashion magazines and helps you appreciate you.*

CHAPTER

2

The Beauty-Brain Loop

The kind of beauty I want most is the hard-to-get kind
that comes from within—strength, courage, dignity.

—Ruby Dee

BACK IN 2007, the Dove company launched a series of ads that received quite a bit of media attention. The women featured in the ads were revolutionary by Madison Avenue agency standards. Instead of emaciated models reflecting some genetic ideal, viewers saw "real" women mostly over age fifty with wide hips, flat chests, skinny legs, gray hair, or even—horrors!—wrinkles. The idea was to portray the company's Pro-Age line of skin-care products as designed to bring out the beauty in any woman of any age.

Sure, this series of TV spots, magazine spreads, and billboards was admirable in drawing attention to the beauty of women who weren't young and perfect. To us, though, as with the Faith Hill brouhaha we mentioned in Chapter 1, the vocal response it engendered seemed out of proportion. It was as if Dorothy had pulled back the curtain on the Great and Powerful Oz to reveal a fifty-two-year-old mother of four from Evanston, Illinois, with spider veins, a dazzling smile, and thinning hair. We assumed a mature nation would say, "Yeah, so what?" Instead, people pointed and exclaimed, "Look! Real women! Honey, you're not going to believe this; come quick!"

The fact remains that these women were really *beautiful.* They weren't runway material, but they all flashed beaming smiles, projected tremendous poise and confidence, and just glowed with self-esteem. They had been chosen to represent their age-group, and they were proud of it. They felt wonderful, and so they looked wonderful. In that way, the campaign was inspiring . . . and a perfect example of how inner beauty evokes outer beauty. That recognition was a long time coming.

INTENTIONALLY BEAUTIFUL

Wellness, health, and beauty are *intentions.* We live in a society where women are still defined by their appearance. Even if you're in your twenties or thirties, this state of affairs can be difficult to accept. You want to be recognized for who you are, not just how you look. Let's face it, if you're gorgeous, it's easier to coast through life knowing that people are going to open doors and do favors for you. However, that's not the path to personal development. Beauty fades with time, and then what do you have left?

Discipline, personal empowerment, and optimism free us from this fate. They really are the elixir of lasting beauty for women of any age. One of life's wonderful balances is that as the years pass, our experience and self-knowledge bloom. Susan Sarandon ages into serene sultriness; Tina Turner goes from has-been abuse victim to sexagenarian sex symbol.

It's possible to reinvent yourself at every level by becoming fully aware of the beauty within you and allowing yourself to cultivate love, confidence, purpose, and compassion. Your inner health will shape your physical self, and you'll be astonished at how the world responds to you.

BECOME A "BLUE LIGHT SPECIAL"

Our goal for this book is simple: come up with a new standard for self-worth that goes beyond physical beauty.

How seismic a shift would that be? Even today, when so many women are leaders in science and industry and shapers of public discourse, we still define ourselves (and allow ourselves to be defined) by our looks. For proof, tune in to your typical television news program. Notice the difference between male and female on-air personalities. It's fine for the men to be gray-haired and "distinguished," but nine times out of ten the female counterparts will be attractive, telegenic eye candy under age forty and wearing figure-hugging ensembles. There's nothing wrong with a female journalist's looking good, but if you scanned the résumés of graduates of the Columbia School of Journalism, we suspect you'd find dozens of women with superior qualifications who went into print or radio because they didn't have the "cute factor."

When you enter a room, you can try *not* to be noticed, or you can go *out of your way* to be noticed. A woman trying to remain invisible glowers at the floor, slumps her shoulders, and doesn't smile. In contrast, the woman whose eyes are animated, whose smile is dazzling, and who walks with a self-assured stride, chin up and shoulders back, shines with a kind of blue light. That's what we call being a "blue light special." It's knowing that you don't just look wonderful but that you also *are* wonderful inside and out, and are not afraid to broadcast it.

BEAUTY STORY: "HELEN"

A successful graphic designer in her forties, Helen came to see Debra for a severe case of eczema—painful, scaly red patches on her face—accompanied by a flaky scalp and acne breakouts on her face and chest. Her family doctor had suggested a ten-day course of steroids to knock the inflammation down, but Helen hated taking any kind of medication and wanted a second opinion. Debra noticed that Helen was a good thirty pounds overweight, and Helen mentioned that she was suffering from chronic insomnia and stress.

Helen shared the fact that since taking a job as art director at a trade publication two years earlier, she had stopped exercising and ate many meals at her desk. She seldom left the office before nine P.M. and had taken to drinking two or three glasses of red wine in the evening to unwind. She felt that her life was "a mess." Previously, as a freelance designer, she made time at least twice a week to take a long hike and devoted at least one day a week to her own art projects. She had enjoyed cooking and never needed to diet to maintain a healthy weight.

After taking a long look at her past choices, Helen took a brave step and decided to return to self-employment. When she did, the other parts of her life began to fall back into place. The red wine turned out to be a trigger for her dermatitis, and the extra weight began to dissolve. Six months later, she looked and felt radiant.

Debra: *Stress triggers a flood of hormones that activate sebaceous activity and sweat, causing an increase in acne. Helen's eczema flare-up was also related to her immune system; stress has a profound impact on the body's ability to protect itself. So, the first step to healing Helen's skin was to encourage her to deal with the causes of her stress.*

Eva: Clearly, she was the victim of too many adrenaline cocktails. The constant deadlines at her job produced a flood of adrenaline, and while some individuals thrive on tension, Helen isn't one of them.

Debra: As she addressed her lifestyle, I created a skin-care regimen for her, a daily program that included a glycolic cleanser to hasten the sloughing of dead skin cells, a topical antibiotic to eliminate the bacteria that trigger eruptions, and a retinol night cream to help her skin regenerate. She also had blue light treatments in my office. In this procedure, a high-intensity, narrow-band blue light is used to treat mild to moderate acne. I was able to target the abnormal bacteria on her skin and decrease her pore size. For Helen's eczema, I recommended that she take shorter, lukewarm showers with an unscented moisturizing soap, followed immediately by an emollient moisturizer. And for her scalp condition, I prescribed a therapeutic shampoo and scalp solution.

You have what it takes to be a drop-dead amazing blue light special right now. Realizing that is half the battle.

WHAT IS THE BEAUTY-BRAIN LOOP?

In that battle, your most reliable weapon is a firm understanding of how mind affects body and vice versa. Your emotional health, self-esteem, and self-confidence shape your physical beauty. At the same time, your health, appearance, and physical well-being affect your state of mind. It's a two-way feedback loop that we call the Beauty-Brain Loop. Beauty does matter, and we aren't ashamed to admit it, but there is so much more to it.

The Beauty-Brain Loop embodies the fundamental physics of magnetism. It is a holistic cycle with four interwoven states:

1. Inner beauty. First is your mental and emotional wellness: self-awareness, self-esteem, and confidence. Inner beauty means constantly taking an honest personal inventory of how you look and how you feel about yourself. It means loving your strengths and accepting your weaknesses, changing what you can and accepting what you cannot. It's your attitude toward the world, your cognitive skills in handling stress, and your ability to see beauty around you.

2. Health. This part of the loop is about taking care of your body from head to toes and from gut to skin. Physical health is shaped by your workout habits, your nutrition, and the amount of nightly sleep you get. It's certainly about how you care for and protect your skin and hair and, without question, how stress impacts your body. Good health is beautiful.

3. Outer beauty. Your appearance is your outer beauty: skin, hair, fitness, clothes, nails, makeup, and more. This is the surface beauty that truly does influence our health, happiness, social station, and success. It's the packaging that both conceals and advertises the woman within.

4. Environment. Nowhere is the power of the Beauty-Brain Loop more obvious than in how your environment responds to you. You can see it all around you: people who feel good not only look good but also are magnetic. The environment falls in line for them. They receive the job offers, get out of traffic tickets, and score the hot table at the restaurant nobody else can even get into. Luck seems to break their way, but it's not luck. It's the power some women and men have to make other people feel good and want to return the favor. Your environment is the reward channel of the loop, and when it's giving you positive feedback, you feel fantastic mentally and physically. We also advocate building a beautiful environment—surrounding yourself with beauty in nature, in your home, and in your relationships.

The loop has no beginning and no end. Each stage affects all the others; everything you do shapes how you feel about yourself and therefore how attractive you are. For example, suppose you have strong self-esteem, due in part to your loving, supportive parents. Even though you're not model material, you like yourself. You're always trying to improve. You're generous. Your **inner beauty** is strong. This shapes your **health**, because you take care of yourself. You love the endorphin high of a workout, so you hit the gym six days a week. You eat wholesome food and love to cook organic meals for friends or even when you're home alone. You wear sunscreen and hydrate, which is a boon for your skin.

As a result, your **outer beauty** surpasses that of other women who might have greater genetic gifts. You're fit. You always dress well and look your best. In conversation, you're smart and witty, and you always ask questions to draw out the other person. Men and women are drawn to you. In turn, you create an **environment** filled with positive feedback. You have a robust dating life and wonderful friends. You're on the upward path at a career you enjoy. You love your life. Your happiness and optimism keep your inner beauty strong, and back around we go. . . .

In the Beauty-Brain Loop, every aspect of your inner and outer life affects every other aspect. How good you feel about your level of physical fitness influences whether you're willing to do cognitive exercises to control your anger. Proper care of your skin can make you see someone more beautiful in the mirror. The interactions are profound and inescapable.

BEAUTY PEARLS

Our idea of beauty was forced to change as women over forty became the most influential consumers in the country. Looking young or replicating a specific ideal is no longer the goal—looking "natural," healthy, fresh, and contemporary is what we're after.

This new concept of mature beauty is driven by the wellness, fitness, and health industries and by celebrities over forty who gave face to the positive imaging of older women. Oscar winners Helen Mirren and Halle Berry, L'Oréal's Diane Keaton and Garnier Nutrisse's Sarah Jessica Parker, Speaker of the House Nancy Pelosi and Senator Hillary Clinton, Madonna, and hundreds more inspire us. Mature women comfortable with their looks, confident in their abilities, and proud of their achievements have created a new definition of beauty—a celebratory approach to age.

The idea of inner/outer beauty has genuine appeal for women over forty, but we're not off the hook maintenance-wise when it comes to looking good. In fact, it takes more effort and strategizing than ever to stay in the game. Daily workouts, devotion to good skin care, wearing a sunscreen of at least SPF 30, and a healthful diet are simply not negotiable. That is the baseline long-term plan no matter what else you choose to do.

Every woman can do the following three things to look better:

*1. **Erase or minimize your cumulative sun damage.** Those brown spots and dull, uneven skin are not looks-friendly. Try over-the-counter products, prescribed skin treatments, or dermatological procedures, from Renova or Retin-A to resurfacing lasers and collagen-boosting creams with antioxidants such as vitamin C and peptides.*

*2. **Update your makeup to sheer, hydrating formulas that give a glow.** A tinted moisturizer, light-reflecting brush-on concealer, tinted lip balm, and cream blush should be in your kit. Add a cream compact foundation for*

> *extra coverage, a rosy nude moisturizing lipstick, and brown/charcoal gel cream liner to enhance definition for work or evenings out.*
>
> *3. Cut your hair sexier and style it healthier. Long bangs and layers camouflage and contemporize every length, while highlights and styling products build texture. Thickening spray, styling cream, and shine spray are essentials. Treat hair like skin, with moisturizing masks, vitamin-enriched serums, and leave-in conditioners to promote healthy hair and scalp.*
>
> —Lois Joy Johnson, beauty and fashion director, More *magazine*

BE MADLY IN LOVE WITH YOURSELF

Mastering the Beauty-Brain Loop puts you in charge not only of how you see yourself but of how others see you as well. However, the loop can also become a vicious cycle. At the same time that it gives you the power to transform your mind and body, it also demands that you stay on top of things, from your weight to your attitude. If there's a link that's not functioning well, the loop works backward. Less attractive people often experience a more negative response from their environment. That can lead to depression and body-damaging behaviors such as overeating, not exercising, or not paying attention to grooming. The negative health consequences of these behaviors usually show up on the skin, affecting outer beauty, and the downward spiral continues.

Even the most genetically blessed women who grew up with highly critical parents or childhood trauma can have impaired inner beauty because of grief or anger. As a result, even if they are physically stunning, their perceptions about how they look and how the environment reacts to them are skewed. They think other people see them as damaged, flawed, or ugly. This leads to unhealthy behaviors and even mental disorders such as body dysmorphic disorder, in which people develop an unhealthy preoccupation with an imagined defect in their appearance. This can lead to poor health and a less attractive appearance.

For true beauty, you've got to balance what's inside with what's outside. We can all gather from the publicized travails of Hollywood's leading ladies that good looks are not a direct link to happiness and a good life. Good looks don't even guarantee you a good relationship. Sure, those looks will open lots of doors and get you lots of dates, but there's so much more that needs to go into a "happily ever after."

It's not a stretch to believe that your physical condition affects your mental state. After all, bad news from the bathroom scale can send some women into a daylong funk. If you doubt that your mind can affect your attractiveness, think about the last time a romantic relationship ended badly. Too often, when that happens and a woman tries to meet someone new, she dresses to the nines and hits the bars looking good, but the guys stay away. Why? She's got the dreaded "D word" tattooed on her forehead: *desperation.*

But when that same woman is in a rewarding relationship, feeling loved and sexy, she's irresistible. What gives? She looks the same; she's the same person; in fact, she probably isn't dressed as well as when she was unattached, because she's not trying to impress anybody. What changed? She did, on the inside. People are typically drawn to others who make them feel good, so when you are smiling, happy, and confident, it's natural for others to be attracted to you. Your positive feelings cause the "feel good" part of their brains to fire, and they want to feel the same way you do.

🌸 BEAUTY BOOSTERS

Practical things you can do now to be more beautiful

Give thought to what you eat and drink. Most of us are chronically dehydrated. We drink soda and coffee, which actually work as diuretics and drain water out of the body. Water, which makes up more than half of a woman's body mass, is constantly being depleted by exercise, heat, and simple respiration. Drink at least eight glasses of water a day to hydrate your body. Also make an effort to include the following foods in your daily diet:

- *Fresh fruits and vegetables, especially berries and brightly colored vegetables rich in antioxidants*

- *Oily fish such as wild salmon and anchovies*

- *Flaxseed and other oils rich in omega-3 fatty acids, such as borage and primrose*

- *Other healthy mono- and polyunsaturated fats such as olive oil and macadamia nut oil*

- *Raw seeds and nuts (full of omega-3s)*

What's good for your heart and your weight is good for your skin and brain. Avoid the bad stuff: refined and processed foods, saturated fats, grease, high-sugar foods, and high-sodium foods.

Need and self-doubt are rarely attractive (except to the wrong person), but display joie de vivre and a little bit of swagger, and you're the center of attention. The trick is to feel positive about yourself as often as possible, whether you're in a relationship or not. When you can be madly in love with yourself under any circumstances, you'll always be beautiful. People will be fascinated by you without even knowing why. Emotions are contagious.

BLURRING THE LINE BETWEEN INSIDE AND OUT

The Beauty-Brain Loop encompasses the deep pathways that transmit information between the mind and the body. You can see this at work in a field called *psychodermatology*. As described by John Koo and Andrew Lebwohl in *American Family Physician*, this science involves how people's mental or emotional state affects the health of their skin, from diseases produced by stress hormones to self-mutilation. Some mind-body experts further suggest that a woman's inner state of being can directly change her appearance.

"People's physical looks actually concretely change depending on their emotional and spiritual condition," says Nancy Scheinman, Ph.D., a mind-body psychologist in Bal Harbour, Florida. "You can have a beautiful woman who looks less than her best because she's not happy. The state of a person's body is a direct outgrowth of what is happening emotionally or what's going on in the person's life. It's a behavioral feedback loop. Your outer appearance is an expression of your inner emotional life."

If you don't believe this, look at yourself first thing in the morning as opposed to when you're excited at the prospect of going out for the evening. We'll bet you look better when you're planning to go out. One of the first signs Eva sees in her patients as they are coming out of their anxiety or depression is that they look better. It may be a small change such as smiling more or better grooming, or a big change such as weight loss after years of hiding behind extra pounds.

BEAUTY BUSTERS

Beauty myths debunked while you wait

Myth: Fear is the main motivator for change.

Fact: You can't sustain lifelong change based on fear. Once the fear fades, you lose your motivation. Fear usually leads to avoidance, so instead of confronting your shortcomings, you end up avoiding situations that make you feel afraid. Don't try to change yourself because you're afraid of getting old or of what other people think of you. You've got to learn to "frame" your reasons for change in a positive, empowering way so that confronting your fears and feeling good becomes a reward. Fear can get you moving, but as soon as the fear enters your mind, make a conscious decision to reframe the fear in a way that's constructive and suggests a positive goal. So, if your doctor tells you that you have high blood pressure, instead of thinking, "Oh my God, I have to get thin or I'm going to have a heart attack!" train yourself to think, "OK, this is a wonderful reason for me to get in shape after all these years and enjoy better health without having to take medication." You'll find that positively motivated change is far more sustainable.

Inner beauty also drives the actions we take to attain our own ideal of beauty, and these actions can be healthful or unhealthful. A healthful example is recognizing that you are important and carving out the time to exercise no matter how many people are pulling at you to do other things. Unhealthful examples include starving yourself, binge eating or purging, using stimulants or laxatives to lose weight, and overexercising. When women are willing to abuse their bodies to look better, something is wrong.

MASTERING THE BEAUTY-BRAIN LOOP

Since each part of the loop affects all the others, taking positive action anywhere channels positive results throughout. The key is doing something, making some positive changes. Get a facial peel that refreshes your skin. Learn to meditate and calm your mind. Hire a personal trainer, and start working out five days a week. Take long walks or long lunches with old friends. Anything you do that makes you feel healthier, more at peace, or more accepting of yourself sends ripples up and down the loop, elevating your inner and outer beauty.

When you take positive steps, your environment rewards you almost immediately. This is why the Beauty-Brain Loop works so well: it gives us control over how the environment reacts to us. If the lifelong quest to look our best is about recapturing control in the face of relentless nature, nothing does this better than being able to determine the effect you have on other people. When you lose weight or overcome social anxiety, people notice. When you look good, feel good, and carry yourself with pride, the environment slaps you a big high-five. Doors open, and people pay attention. It's life-affirming and fantastic. We encourage you to try it!

THE CONFIDENCE PARADOX

When you get to the point where your beauty is eliciting consistent positive feedback from your environment, you exemplify the "confidence paradox." It's a secret that we're going to let you in on.

The paradox works like this: Most of us base our self-assessment of how we look on comparisons with the people around us. Studies have shown that when women are around other women who meet the typical physical standard for beauty—young, slender, and blonde—they feel less attractive. UC Davis psychologist Richard Robins attests in *Psychology Today* that women tend to evaluate their physical attractiveness by comparing themselves with an idealized version of beauty, usually a fashion model. For some reason, we don't compare our IQ with Einstein's; we're more realistic. But in our YouTube and twenty-four-hour cable society, we are relentlessly bombarded with images of extraordinarily attractive young women. These images make us feel worse about ourselves.

On the upside, as our environment—our employment situation, social circle, and romantic life—begins to reward us for self-improvement, we free our minds from harmful comparisons with others and start feeling and being better. We sit in a public place and watch "real" women pass and realize we look pretty good. We begin to shine with self-confidence even when confronted with size-zero fashion models and objectifying stereotypes. That makes us even more attractive.

That's the confidence paradox. When you're overly concerned about what other people think of your appearance, your insecu-

---

BEAUTY PEARLS

I think a woman is most beautiful when she breaks into a full smile and you can tell that the smile also comes from within.

—Amy Hendel, RPA, health journalist,
"Today Show" contributor, iVillage blogger and coach,
family lifestyle therapist, and author of Fat Families, Thin Families

rity and self-doubt make you less attractive, whereas when you *know* that you look and feel fabulous regardless of how you stack up against anybody else, your attractiveness and magnetism skyrocket. If the only one you try to impress is *you*, you'll impress everyone else as well!

WORKING THE LOOP WITH OTHER WOMEN

You don't have to impress anyone at the salon, and that's what makes it wonderful. The idea of the salon is appealing not just as a place to get hair and nails done but also in its old European definition as a place to gather and carry on civilized conversation. That's what we would like to see the salon become for women: a place where we can gather to give each other love and support and share bits of our lives while getting facials and pedicures. There are so few places in our society where women can just get together and spend time. Women are social creatures, and we need these opportunities to feel pampered in a girls' club environment. By nurturing ourselves and others, we are stimulating those feel-good endorphins and becoming more healthy and beautiful.

Try to surround yourself with people who think highly of you and give you positive feedback on how you look. If you're always in the company of people who are demeaning or overly sexual, you're going to have problems with your self-esteem. It is impossible to tune out others completely. How you're treated impacts your self-image. So, every woman needs a place that can be an oasis, where women celebrate each other's whole beauty, inside and out. Working the Beauty-Brain Loop can be done best with some assistance, whether from your dermatologist, therapist, hairdresser, or best friend.

There Are No Victims

The Dutch medical ethicist Medard T. Hilhorst writes that a person's attractiveness depends on many features appreciated at many levels:

- Physical looks (body, face, figure)
- Artistic looks (clothes, makeup, perfume, hair)
- Personal looks (appearance, impression, aura)
- Performance (voice, attitude, behavior)
- Personality (charm, charisma, appeal, allure)
- Relational capacities (the ability to communicate and make a connection)
- Friendship abilities (reliability, spontaneity, warmth, empathy, caring)

How many of those items are beyond your control? Exactly none. Every aspect of personal attractiveness is within your ability to change, if that is what you want. You are not the victim of your DNA. There are no victims; there are only women who haven't realized their power yet. You don't have to spend your life averting your eyes from the magazines at the supermarket checkout aisle. Instead of reacting to your environment, you can use the Beauty-Brain Loop to decide how the environment will react to *you*.

But first, a little self-awareness is in order. We hope you've been paying attention, because it's time for a "faith lift."

Beauty Bullets

ↄ Beauty is an intention.

ↄ The Beauty-Brain Loop gives you the power to transcend your biology and make yourself more beautiful.

ↄ Your state of mind affects your physical appearance in many ways.

ↄ If you're confident enough not to worry about what others think, they'll find you impossible to resist.

ↄ Self-actualized women are the most beautiful.

BEAUTY AND THE BRAIN Rx

Your Foundation

Dr. Debra: Hydrate your skin. It's the simplest way to keep it healthy. Decrease your exposure to hot water, caffeine, and public enemy number one: the sun. Drink six to eight glasses of water a day, and start taking luke-warm showers. When you get out of the shower, don't dry off completely— apply a moisturizer directly to your hydrated skin, preferably one with a mineral oil base or that contains an alpha hydroxy acid. This way, your skin should be well hydrated for twenty-four hours.

Dr. Eva: Think of your own mentors and role models who have the greatest inner beauty. What qualities do they have that you would like to emulate? Make a list of those qualities and assess which ones need the most work.

Now assign yourself three things you can do that will improve each. At the same time, keep doing the positive things you are already doing. Always strengthen the positive while improving the negative. That may mean continuing to do charity work while going to therapy. Each one of us is a work in progress, and it is up to us to decide which aspects of ourselves we want to improve and which we can feel wonderful about already.

3

The Beauty Prescription Quiz

The best vision is insight.

—Malcolm Forbes

CONSIDER BARBIE. SHE'S got quite the life. First of all, she's built like a Greek goddess. She's got castles, Corvettes, and beach houses. She's got cool friends such as Skipper and a handsome-yet-sensitive boyfriend, Ken, who never asks for a commitment. With that package of attributes going for her, Barbie has become part of our pop-culture mythos. Songs are written about her. She's the main playmate of millions of young girls and has been for more than forty years. Like it or not, the Mattel temptress has become something of a feminine ideal.

To explore that phenomenon, a group of Canadian media researchers generated a computer model of a woman with Barbie's "generous" measurements and found that her back would be too weak to support the weight of her well-endowed upper body, and her emaciated torso would be too narrow to hold more than half a liver and a few inches of colon. If she were a real woman, they concluded, Barbie would eventually die from malnutrition.

THE CULT OF BARBIE

Poor Barbie. Behind the smiling facade, doomed by her tiny gastrointestinal tract. It should be obvious from one look that these are not the proportions of a real human being, but that doesn't stop millions of women, young and old, from wanting to look like her. The influence of the "cult of Barbie" can be seen in the spread of eating disorders and in "tween" girls begging their parents for breast augmentation surgery at a time when they should be getting worked up about Hello Kitty backpacks.

BEAUTY PEARLS

Beauty comes from the inside and radiates out. This is the basic concept of shen, the waking consciousness that makes us human. My mother drilled the saying "beauty is what beauty does" into me, and it is paramount to me as a mother, woman, and role model to my patients to be kind and beautiful from the inside. I have spent an enormous amount of time with the most beautiful women and men in the world, and the ugliness that emanated from most of them was shocking.

I truly practice what I preach. I meditate every day. I am a food purist and attempt to feed my family the same way. I work out every day, and, most of all, I stay grateful and humble for the truly wonderful people, patients, friends, and family in my life.

—Elizabeth Trattner, former model,
nationally board-certified doctor of Chinese medicine

Would-be Barbies fall into two major types. The first is actually trying to achieve perfection but is unwittingly wrecking her health and her looks in doing so. These women yo-yo diet, have unnecessary cosmetic surgery, and spend a fortune on unproven products. The second type isn't even giving a thought to her health or beauty; she's just letting herself go without grasping the price she'll pay in ten or twenty years.

The purpose of the Beauty Prescription Quiz is to help every woman, cultists and noncultists alike, become aware not just of what she's doing right but also of the ways in which she's denying herself her birthright—to be attractive, magnetic, and marvelous—through poor habits, deficient self-esteem, or ill-advised choices. It's a master's degree course in yourself.

DIVING INTO YOUR DEEPEST END

The preceding chapters presented examples of the ways we fool ourselves into thinking magazine and television images are real people whom we can emulate. Trying to do this is inevitably self-defeating, because the images are two-dimensional. Mirrors are the same, which is why they can't help but lie. It's impossible to convey real attractiveness in two dimensions; that's why retouching is the norm. No photo or video footage will ever do you justice. You're multidimensional. No image can capture your personality or passion. For the same reason, "fixing things" by getting emergency liposuction or breast enhancement makes no sense. You're fixing only one dimension. That's shallow. You're a woman of deep feeling and complexity. In fact, you have depths you probably don't even know.

In the quiz, we're going to plumb those depths. We're going to ask you a lot of questions, and we urge you to answer them with the utmost honesty. You owe that to yourself. You might think you know a lot about your inner and outer beauty; after all, you're the expert on you. But it's what you *don't* know (or haven't admitted) that's going to make all the difference. You're going to discover the areas in which you're strong as well as ones in which you need improvement without delay.

Honest answers and the willingness to gain new insights are the means to making the four pieces of the Beauty-Brain Loop work together. Remember that each stage affects all the others. Without knowing what you're doing wrong in each stage and taking the proper remedial steps, you're like an engine that's misfiring on a cylinder.

As physicians, we're accustomed to obtaining complete medical histories from our patients. Because they come to our offices, we have the opportunity to ask them a battery of questions and learn details about their lives that can give us clues as to how to help them. Obviously, we can't do that with you, but that doesn't mean we can't get at information that helps. You just need to do the gathering. Then in the following chapters, we'll share our experience and knowledge in ways that will help you turn the insights you gain from the quiz into constructive action that enhances your beauty and your life.

An Act of Faith

Chapter 2 concluded by planting the idea of a "faith lift." The quiz requires having sufficient faith to be candid about your answers and to accept any results that might seem discouraging and turn them into action. It's a stripping away of the illusions we've been talking about—cosmetic surgery for the soul. As with

BEAUTY BUDDIES

Anna Lefler, stand-up comedian and writer, forty-three; Dori Andrunas, full-time mom, forty-two

Anna and Dori have been close friends for almost twenty years, since they met in graduate school. They are alike in many ways: similar professional, educational, and cultural backgrounds as well as similar views about beauty, taste, elegance, and gracefully holding their ground against the encroachment of time on their bodies and psyches.

"I think we're ideal Beauty Buddies because we know each other so well and have so much in common," says Anna, a stand-up comedian and budding author. "We swap information about new treatments, products, and procedures without competition or agenda. Because we're so comfortable and accepting of one another, we can talk openly about the things we like about our appearances and the things we'd like to improve. We can also tell each other to lighten up when we get too self-critical."

Because they live more than an hour apart and both have young children, slipping away for a quick manicure isn't an option. So the heart of Anna and Dori's Beauty Buddies experience is their annual Palm Springs getaway. "Each summer for two or three nights," Anna explains, "we head out to the desert with another close friend or two and really pull the plug on our everyday lives. We try a new spa on each visit, each more decadent than the last. I love trying the most unusual treatments on the menu, while Dori tends to go for the facial and straightforward deep-tissue massage to work out the stresses of everyday life. We also love sitting in the sauna talking about the developments in our lives, sharing our ups and downs, and offering support, advice, congratulations, and condolences. Back at the

(continued)

rental house, the talking continues as we drift around the pool or boil in the hot tub (in between sunscreen applications, of course)."

Anna insists that the benefits of this time go light-years beyond just the cosmetic primping. "The sharing and camaraderie that come from the experience are priceless. Dori and I look forward to this getaway all year long and the little traditions of the experience [revisiting the same restaurants and shops] are important to us. I also think it's comforting to compare notes with my close friends about the changes we're all going through as we age. The little surprises that I see in the mirror in the morning are not quite as discouraging when I can commiserate and laugh about them with my girl-friends who are having similar experiences."

any surgery, there may be some discomfort, but with time comes recovery and new possibility. By facing up to any self-deceptions or negative perceptions of your own beauty that you have been harboring, you restore your confidence in your ability to deal with reality. You don't need to airbrush the world. You can look at yourself as you are, proclaim, "That's all right," and then point yourself in the right direction.

You've encountered your share of beauty quizzes in innumerable health, fitness, style, and beauty magazines, but you haven't seen anything like this. The goal of the Beauty Prescription Quiz is to find out not just how you take care of your skin but also how well you know and love yourself—to help you know where you stand today in your journey toward being a radiant, multidimensional woman. It's not possible to bring about positive change in your inner or outer self without self-awareness, so the quiz is built to help you develop that awareness. Then, with your illusions washed away and your eyes open, you can begin a makeover for your mind and identity, something light-years beyond simply getting your crow's-feet done.

Some parts of the quiz may make you uncomfortable. You will come upon questions whose answers you'd rather not face. We encourage you to face them anyway. Those questions are your opportunities for growth. Only when we see ourselves clearly can we find the necessary motivation to make positive change. Trust us: the truth is never as bad as our fears make it seem. Remember, even Faith Hill isn't perfect. You don't have to be perfect. Just be a resilient, self-confident, fully conscious you. Hang on tight. You're about to take yourself off autopilot. Enjoy the ride.

EYES ON YOUR OWN PAPER!

The format of the quiz is based on the four stages of the Beauty-Brain Loop: Inner Beauty, Health, Outer Beauty, and Environment. For each statement, circle the appropriate number to rate your attitude on a 1–5 scale:

1—You disagree completely with the statement.
2—You disagree somewhat with the statement.
3—You're neutral on or unsure about the statement.
4—You agree somewhat with the statement.
5—You agree completely with the statement.

At the end of each section, we'll ask you to total your score. Then at the end of the quiz, you'll find out what your total score means. So, have at it. And remember, the more open you are, even to uncomfortable truths, the more you will benefit.

Section 1: Inner Beauty

Everything begins here. The mind affects the body. The mind shapes your behavior and self-care. Your confidence and self-esteem can make you ravishing or cowering. Time to know where you stand.

1. My inner voice tends to be positive and optimistic.

   COMPLETELY DISAGREE   1   2   3   4   5   COMPLETELY AGREE

2. When things go wrong in my life, I try not to take it personally. Stuff happens.

   COMPLETELY DISAGREE   1   2   3   4   5   COMPLETELY AGREE

3. When I look in the mirror, I like what I see.

   COMPLETELY DISAGREE   1   2   3   4   5   COMPLETELY AGREE

4. I am comfortable in situations even when I have to be the center of attention.

   COMPLETELY DISAGREE   1   2   3   4   5   COMPLETELY AGREE

5. When I am completely myself, people tend to like me, quirks and all.

   COMPLETELY DISAGREE   1   2   3   4   5   COMPLETELY AGREE

6. I try not to compare my achievements with those of others.

   COMPLETELY DISAGREE   1   2   3   4   5   COMPLETELY AGREE

7. When bad things happen, I take a deep breath and find ways to cope.

   COMPLETELY DISAGREE   1   2   3   4   5   COMPLETELY AGREE

8. I'm not a worrier.

   COMPLETELY DISAGREE   1   2   3   4   5   COMPLETELY AGREE

9. I have a strong spiritual side that I cherish and nurture.

   COMPLETELY DISAGREE   1   2   3   4   5   COMPLETELY AGREE

10. When I go out, I feel confident that people will find me attractive, even if I don't look perfect.

    COMPLETELY DISAGREE   1   2   3   4   5   COMPLETELY AGREE

11. I have a great deal of empathy for the feelings of others.

    COMPLETELY DISAGREE   1   2   3   4   5   COMPLETELY AGREE

12. My intellect and sense of humor are my best features.

    COMPLETELY DISAGREE   1   2   3   4   5   COMPLETELY AGREE

13. I don't care if people gossip about me; the only opinions that matter are those of people I care about.

    COMPLETELY DISAGREE   1   2   3   4   5   COMPLETELY AGREE

14. I'm a habitually upbeat, positive person. I usually don't get the blues.

    COMPLETELY DISAGREE   1   2   3   4   5   COMPLETELY AGREE

15. I feel pleased with the choices I have made in my life, and if some choices haven't worked out, I'm not afraid to admit it and make changes.

COMPLETELY DISAGREE   1   2   3   4   5   COMPLETELY AGREE

16. I practice yoga, meditate, or do something else to manage stress.

COMPLETELY DISAGREE   1   2   3   4   5   COMPLETELY AGREE

BEAUTY STORY: "LESLIE"

Leslie, twenty-four, had been dating a guy for two years, but he had just broken up with her. Leslie said he left her because she had big hips. She was crushed and came into Debra's office insisting that she needed liposuction "this week." Seeing the red flags go up, Debra told Leslie that she thought she had issues that could not be addressed by cosmetic surgery. Leslie left the office upset. A few weeks later, however, she called Debra and thanked her for not doing the liposuction.

Debra: *Contrast Leslie's story with that of another patient of mine, named Becky, a thirty-five-year-old woman who looks good, is in good health, and recently got a promotion and a raise. She had thought about hip liposuction for years; she had tried dieting and exercising, with only limited success. Finally, with her increased income, she had the money for the procedure and felt it was a perfect "finishing touch" for her, so she got the liposuction and loved the results. She felt freer to wear stylish clothing that showed off her new figure.*

Eva: *Becky and Leslie illustrate the difference between healthy, realistic expectations of a surgical intervention and unrealistic ones, such as thinking you're going to get your boyfriend back by sculpting your body.*

17. I don't care if other people don't "get" me; what I think about myself matters most.

    COMPLETELY DISAGREE 1 2 3 4 5 COMPLETELY AGREE

18. I am grateful for the opportunities in my life.

    COMPLETELY DISAGREE 1 2 3 4 5 COMPLETELY AGREE

19. My first thought in any difficult situation is, "What can I do to make this better?"

    COMPLETELY DISAGREE 1 2 3 4 5 COMPLETELY AGREE

20. My self-esteem is very strong.

    COMPLETELY DISAGREE 1 2 3 4 5 COMPLETELY AGREE

Your total score: _____ out of a possible 100.

Section 2: Health

How much you love yourself, as well as what habits you acquired during childhood and beyond, will dictate how well you take care of yourself. Your fitness, diet, health care, and skin care are all in play.

21. I get at least one hour of strenuous exercise three to five days a week.

    COMPLETELY DISAGREE 1 2 3 4 5 COMPLETELY AGREE

22. I lift weights in a regular program or do other muscle-strengthening workouts.

    COMPLETELY DISAGREE 1 2 3 4 5 COMPLETELY AGREE

23. I leave my car at home and walk places or take stairs instead of the elevator.

    COMPLETELY DISAGREE 1 2 3 4 5 COMPLETELY AGREE

24. When I feel tired at the start or end of the day, or just feel down, I work out.

    COMPLETELY DISAGREE 1 2 3 4 5 COMPLETELY AGREE

25. I do yoga, Pilates, or something else to keep my muscles loose and joints flexible.

    COMPLETELY DISAGREE 1 2 3 4 5 COMPLETELY AGREE

26. I do my best to avoid fast or processed food even when I am busy.

    COMPLETELY DISAGREE 1 2 3 4 5 COMPLETELY AGREE

27. I eat three to five servings of fruit and vegetables every day.

    COMPLETELY DISAGREE 1 2 3 4 5 COMPLETELY AGREE

28. I keep my brain stimulated with puzzles, reading, and challenging conversation.

    COMPLETELY DISAGREE 1 2 3 4 5 COMPLETELY AGREE

29. I drink at least eight glasses of water every day.

    COMPLETELY DISAGREE 1 2 3 4 5 COMPLETELY AGREE

30. I take at least a multivitamin/mineral supplement daily.

    COMPLETELY DISAGREE 1 2 3 4 5 COMPLETELY AGREE

31. I have an annual physical.

COMPLETELY DISAGREE 1 2 3 4 5 COMPLETELY AGREE

32. I get an annual Pap smear.

COMPLETELY DISAGREE 1 2 3 4 5 COMPLETELY AGREE

33. I know my blood pressure and cholesterol count.

COMPLETELY DISAGREE 1 2 3 4 5 COMPLETELY AGREE

34. I get enough sleep most nights, usually six to eight hours.

COMPLETELY DISAGREE 1 2 3 4 5 COMPLETELY AGREE

35. I am a nonsmoker.

COMPLETELY DISAGREE 1 2 3 4 5 COMPLETELY AGREE

36. I don't believe in crash dieting, because the weight loss is always temporary.

COMPLETELY DISAGREE 1 2 3 4 5 COMPLETELY AGREE

37. Whenever I go out in the sun, I use a sunscreen with at least SPF 15 that protects against both UVA and UVB rays.

COMPLETELY DISAGREE 1 2 3 4 5 COMPLETELY AGREE

38. If I drink alcohol, it's usually no more than one glass of wine in an evening.

COMPLETELY DISAGREE 1 2 3 4 5 COMPLETELY AGREE

39. I'm within ten pounds of my ideal weight.

COMPLETELY DISAGREE   1   2   3   4   5   COMPLETELY AGREE

40. Dental care is important; I see my dentist twice a year like clockwork.

COMPLETELY DISAGREE   1   2   3   4   5   COMPLETELY AGREE

Your total score: _____ out of a possible 100.

BEAUTY BOOSTERS

Practical things you can do now to be more beautiful

The saying "The eyes are the windows to the soul" is true. Your eyes communicate your emotions like no other part of your face. For instance, a Boston College psychologist showed that the stress levels of political candidates during televised debates correlated to the rate at which they blinked. Your eyes reveal much about you—fatigue, fear, aging, happiness, flirtatiousness, joy, anger.

So, it's important that you care for your eyes. Circles under the eyes are generally caused by an increase in skin pigment or in the visibility of veins, due to either genetics or inflammation. Deeply set eyes make circles even more prominent. To reduce circles, use cold compresses of green tea bags. These help alleviate vascular congestion and are also anti-inflammatory. Then use an eye cream with hyaluronic acid, which will hydrate sunken eyes and decrease the appearance of crow's-feet. Allergies are a common cause of dark circles and should be treated.

Section 3: Outer Beauty

Surface counts too. What do you do to maximize your outer beauty? This section is devoted to your grooming, clothing, and overall appearance.

41. I use a nonabrasive exfoliant a few times a week.

    COMPLETELY DISAGREE   1   2   3   4   5   COMPLETELY AGREE

42. I always remove my makeup before I go to bed.

    COMPLETELY DISAGREE   1   2   3   4   5   COMPLETELY AGREE

43. I put on a broad-spectrum sunscreen whenever I'm going to be in the sun for more than a few minutes.

    COMPLETELY DISAGREE   1   2   3   4   5   COMPLETELY AGREE

44. I keep up on fashion trends, but I wear only what I like. I don't need to look like a magazine cover.

    COMPLETELY DISAGREE   1   2   3   4   5   COMPLETELY AGREE

45. I would have a cosmetic procedure only if it were something I wanted. I would never have it to please somebody else.

    COMPLETELY DISAGREE   1   2   3   4   5   COMPLETELY AGREE

46. I have a great smile.

    COMPLETELY DISAGREE   1   2   3   4   5   COMPLETELY AGREE

47. I keep my nails healthy and groomed.

    COMPLETELY DISAGREE   1   2   3   4   5   COMPLETELY AGREE

48. My hairstyle accentuates my best features while camouflaging my weakest.

COMPLETELY DISAGREE 1 2 3 4 5 COMPLETELY AGREE

49. If I gain a couple of pounds, I don't beat myself up about it.

COMPLETELY DISAGREE 1 2 3 4 5 COMPLETELY AGREE

50. I have cosmetics and makeup that really work for me.

COMPLETELY DISAGREE 1 2 3 4 5 COMPLETELY AGREE

51. I know how to use makeup in a way that accentuates my best features.

COMPLETELY DISAGREE 1 2 3 4 5 COMPLETELY AGREE

52. I can get ready quickly if I need to.

COMPLETELY DISAGREE 1 2 3 4 5 COMPLETELY AGREE

53. I'm good at accessorizing—never too much or too little.

COMPLETELY DISAGREE 1 2 3 4 5 COMPLETELY AGREE

54. I am proud of my posture and know it makes me more attractive.

COMPLETELY DISAGREE 1 2 3 4 5 COMPLETELY AGREE

55. I know how to dress appropriately for my age while looking classy and attractive.

COMPLETELY DISAGREE 1 2 3 4 5 COMPLETELY AGREE

56. I try to wear clothes that put my best foot forward. I know the strengths and weaknesses of my body type and have figured out what is most flattering on me.

    COMPLETELY DISAGREE 1 2 3 4 5 COMPLETELY AGREE

57. Other women often say to me, "You have to tell me where you got that!"

    COMPLETELY DISAGREE 1 2 3 4 5 COMPLETELY AGREE

58. I enjoy putting myself together for any event, from a football game to a formal dinner.

    COMPLETELY DISAGREE 1 2 3 4 5 COMPLETELY AGREE

59. I always make time for the beauty salon.

    COMPLETELY DISAGREE 1 2 3 4 5 COMPLETELY AGREE

60. I keep my beauty regimen simple: a handful of products that I know work for me.

    COMPLETELY DISAGREE 1 2 3 4 5 COMPLETELY AGREE

Your total score: _____ out of a possible 100.

Section 4: Environment

Your surroundings have an impact on your inner and outer beauty. Your environment is everyone and everything around you; it's all responding to how you look, how you feel, and how you carry yourself.

61. I have a private sanctuary in my home where I can go to relax completely.

    COMPLETELY DISAGREE   1   2   3   4   5   COMPLETELY AGREE

62. I enjoy meeting new people.

    COMPLETELY DISAGREE   1   2   3   4   5   COMPLETELY AGREE

63. I'm the kind of person who knows people wherever I go.

    COMPLETELY DISAGREE   1   2   3   4   5   COMPLETELY AGREE

64. I put myself in different environments to make sure I am always stimulated.

    COMPLETELY DISAGREE   1   2   3   4   5   COMPLETELY AGREE

65. I have a wonderful support network of friends or family who accept me as I am.

    COMPLETELY DISAGREE   1   2   3   4   5   COMPLETELY AGREE

66. I try to nurture relationships through the years. As the saying goes, make new friends and keep the old.

    COMPLETELY DISAGREE   1   2   3   4   5   COMPLETELY AGREE

67. I am happy in my current dating or marital situation.

    COMPLETELY DISAGREE   1   2   3   4   5   COMPLETELY AGREE

68. I have someone with whom I can be open and share everything.

    COMPLETELY DISAGREE   1   2   3   4   5   COMPLETELY AGREE

69. I don't feel threatened when I am surrounded by beautiful women in person or in the media.

COMPLETELY DISAGREE 1 2 3 4 5 COMPLETELY AGREE

70. I keep my closet organized so I can find what I need to look and feel my best.

COMPLETELY DISAGREE 1 2 3 4 5 COMPLETELY AGREE

71. I have hobbies that I truly enjoy.

COMPLETELY DISAGREE 1 2 3 4 5 COMPLETELY AGREE

72. I would rather be with people in person than chat on the Internet.

COMPLETELY DISAGREE 1 2 3 4 5 COMPLETELY AGREE

73. I love what fills my days, whether it's a career, school, or raising my kids.

COMPLETELY DISAGREE 1 2 3 4 5 COMPLETELY AGREE

74. I am lucky enough to spend most of my time engaging in activities I enjoy.

COMPLETELY DISAGREE 1 2 3 4 5 COMPLETELY AGREE

75. Good people just seem to show up in my life.

COMPLETELY DISAGREE 1 2 3 4 5 COMPLETELY AGREE

76. I strike a balance between work time and time for family or just caring for myself.

COMPLETELY DISAGREE 1 2 3 4 5 COMPLETELY AGREE

77. I have a place to exercise that really works for me.

COMPLETELY DISAGREE   1   2   3   4   5   COMPLETELY AGREE

78. I always find time to do charitable work or give back to others in meaningful ways.

COMPLETELY DISAGREE   1   2   3   4   5   COMPLETELY AGREE

79. I see beauty around me every day in the most unexpected places.

COMPLETELY DISAGREE   1   2   3   4   5   COMPLETELY AGREE

80. I'm able to stop and live in the moment.

COMPLETELY DISAGREE   1   2   3   4   5   COMPLETELY AGREE

Your total score: _____ out of a possible 100.

OK, Pencils Down!

How did you do? Did you find most of the questions easy, or did you have to do some serious soul-searching? We hope you found at least some of them challenging and thought-provoking and that you answered honestly. No one should score 100! The first time we took this quiz, we were surprised by some of our responses.

We could have asked a hundred more questions about exercise, emotional health, grooming, and all the rest, but then we would have a quiz so long that no one would ever complete it. These eighty questions are intended to give you a reliable picture of your current state in each of the four areas in the Beauty-Brain Loop. Until you know where you are, you can't make plans to get where you want to be.

BEAUTY BUSTERS

Beauty myths debunked while you wait

Myth: Adults cannot change after a certain age.

Fact: This is just an excuse for not being willing to do the heavy lifting of personal transformation. Change can be hard, scary, and painful, but it's possible no matter how old you are. The brain has a profound ability to alter itself, a quality neuroscientists call neuroplasticity. Basically, this means that new thoughts and new experiences actually physically change the brain, creating new neural pathways that replace worn-out ones. Science has also found that no matter how old you are, your brain can create new neural connections. So, there really never is a dog too old to learn new tricks. There are only dogs who won't get off the couch, quit spending time with dogs who criticize their fur, and stop eating table scraps. The changes we're talking about in this chapter are possible. We have seen women of all ages transform their lives.

Of course, we know what you really want right now: to learn how you did on the quiz. First, please understand that there are no right or wrong answers. There's just you. Clearly, we designed the quiz to reveal attitudes and lifestyles we consider healthy or unhealthy, but that doesn't mean there's something wrong with you if you scored poorly on one section. It just means that according to our judgment as physicians and women, there are changes you can and perhaps should make in order to become healthier, more attractive, and happier. Ultimately, that's the universal goal: happiness in bodies and minds that we love and treat as treasures. So . . . let's score the Beauty Prescription Quiz.

Assuming that the best answer for each question is a 5, for "Completely Agree," each set of twenty questions has a perfect total of 100. How well you did in each section depends on how far your score is from 100.

Scoring the Quiz

80–100 in a section: This is a great score. This area is obviously one of your strengths. You might have some work to do, but probably not much.

60–79: This is an OK scoring range. You have many strengths, but there are obviously some things you'd like to improve on. Knowing what needs work is what this book is about.

59 or below: You can really benefit from our chapter devoted to this stage of the Beauty-Brain Loop. Yes, you need some help in this area, but you have help. We're here to advise you on affirmative measures you can take now.

WHAT THE QUIZ MEANS

Surprised by your scores in the quiz? Encouraged? Confused? That's all right; they're all legitimate responses. The most significant reaction you can have to the Beauty Prescription Quiz is to be open-minded.

Our hope is that the quiz will help you start being more truthful with yourself about the areas of your physical and mental health that could be better—to be more self-aware, not only about what's happened in your past but also in real time, throughout your day. If you're committed to changing your habits and lifestyle choices so that you become a more radiant, joyous woman, then you've got to do more than simply look back and say, "Hmm, that was a mistake. I won't do that again." You must also have the awareness to catch yourself when you're over-reacting to a stress situation or choosing to eat junk food, and say, "Stop! This isn't the new, more beautiful me." Remember that perfection is not the goal either, so if you veer off course a bit, that may be OK too. The objective is for the majority of your choices to take you in the right direction—not every choice.

Chances are, you scored pretty well in at least two of the four categories, so-so in another, and lower in a fourth. Everyone has weak areas. We've put you through the quiz to help you priori-tize—to know which stage of the Beauty-Brain Loop you should be working on first. As we said, the loop has no beginning and no end, and each stage affects all the others. So, if your Outer Beauty score was the lowest, that's an ideal place to start, per-haps by looking at your skin care, wardrobe, or grooming. You begin a skin-care regimen, and you start taking on a glow you didn't have before. People notice. This affects your confidence (Inner Beauty) but also prompts you to work out and lose weight (Health). You begin to look better, feel better, and be better. Your self-esteem gets a shot in the arm, and before you know it, people are getting whiplash while watching you enter a confer-ence room. See how it works?

In the end, the quiz is a tool for getting a handle on a ques-tion that can seem despairingly overwhelming: "How do I change my life?" The answer is, you don't. You change a few manageable things at a time, things that snowball and affect other areas. Before you know it, a few changes turn into a sys-temic transformation of your body or your attitude. The key is to know what areas to change to have the greatest effect. It's like pulling a keystone out of a pile of rocks in order to create an ava-lanche. We're going to help you find your keystone—then step back and watch the avalanche of attractiveness and magnetism that you create.

Into the Loop

The four stages of the Beauty-Brain Loop are a kind of personal ecosystem. You can't tweak one part without seeing changes—sometimes unintended—in all the others. Learn all you can, and when you're done with this book, go back and review the quiz and the stage of the loop where you scored the lowest. That's where your work should begin. Of course, do whatever you can in all four stages, especially if you can make pleasurable, easy changes that yield quick results. On the other hand, if you address mild problems with your health by putting in more time at the gym but still have serious shortcomings in terms of self-esteem, pessimism, and ability to trust others, you're just going to spin your wheels. Make progress wherever you can, but hone in on where it's needed most.

All right. Time to get down to business. Let's move on to Part 2 and take an in-depth look at each stage of the Beauty-Brain Loop.

Beauty Bullets

- Barbie may be an icon of beauty, but she's an unhealthy, impossible icon.

- Two-dimensional images cannot capture the beauty of a multidimensional woman.

- Being honest with yourself is the most important aspect of the Beauty Prescription Quiz.

  You should start your changes in the area of the Beauty-Brain Loop where you scored the lowest.

  Progress in one stage of the loop will improve the other stages.

  Take pride in the areas in which you scored high.

 ## BEAUTY AND THE BRAIN Rx

Essentials

Dr. Eva: *Take a look at your quiz results. Which is your strongest area? If your Inner Beauty score is better than your Outer Beauty score, it's time to get gorgeous! Start looking around. Attractive women are everywhere, and you can learn from watching them. On the other hand, if your Outer Beauty is higher than your Inner Beauty, begin the journey of self-love by writing a love letter to yourself. If your Health score is out of balance, see an internist and have a complete medical exam. Inner and Outer Beauty depend on obtaining optimal health. Is your environment bringing you down? List five ways you can improve your environment. Take small, simple steps that will yield quick rewards.*

Dr. Debra: *If your Outer Beauty score is low, you may want to start with a few simple activities. Visit a dermatologist and begin a skin-care routine of cleansers, exfoliation, and sunscreen. My philosophy with skin care is "less is more." You need only a handful of products. Here's my prescription:*

1. In the morning, use a gentle, nonabrasive exfoliating cleanser to remove dead skin cells.

(continued)

2. Every day, apply a physical sunblock, such as zinc oxide, or broad-spectrum sunscreen. That means an SPF of at least 15–30 that may include UVA-stabilizing ingredients such as Mexoryl or Helioplex for maximum UVA and UVB protection. If you live in a place where the sun is more intense, such as a desert or at high elevation, use SPF 30–45 instead.

3. In the evening, use a night cream with an active ingredient such as glycolic acid, antioxidants, or a retinol to shrink pores, increase skin-cell regeneration, and soften fine lines.

Living the Beauty-Brain Loop

4

Inner Beauty: It All Begins Here

Taking joy in living is a woman's best cosmetic.
—Rosalind Russell

ONE OF THE biggest television hits of 2006 was an ABC program with the surprising title "Ugly Betty." The sometimes-outlandish comedic soap opera chronicles the life of a sweet, homely Latina with a mouthful of braces as she tries to fit into the world of high fashion. What we find refreshing about the show is that it's not trying to win viewers by serving up eye candy. The main character is portrayed as unattractive (although away from the show, star America Ferrera is beautiful) but sincere, kind, and genuine—everything her fashion-maven colleagues are supposedly not.

"Ugly Betty" has become one of TV's breakout hits based not on glamour or special effects, but on the inner beauty of its star. Despite all the beautiful faces and exposed skin on dozens of other programs, the one about the frumpy girl makes more people smile, watch, and relate. Betty has inner beauty, and that's its power.

WHAT IS INNER BEAUTY?

Inner beauty is where true beauty begins. At its heart is *self-esteem*. That term is overused and often misunderstood. The dictionary defines it like this:

Realistic respect for or favorable impression of oneself; self-respect.

Self-esteem doesn't come from being given something on a silver platter. The foundation for self-esteem is laid in childhood by the messages we get from our parents and other trusted adults. As we mature, we are more in control of our self-esteem, and we can make efforts to improve it when needed. Nothing is more vital for a healthy mind and a strong sense of beauty.

Let's break the term down to see what's really involved. First, it's about yourself. It's your personal view of yourself. It's how you feel when you are alone with your thoughts. Esteem reflects how valuable you consider yourself to be. Do you hold yourself in high esteem? Do you have self-love, self-acceptance, and self-respect? When you have strong self-esteem, you accept and love all the parts of you. You know you have flaws that may need work, but you are confident in your ability to improve. You understand that nobody is perfect but that you can be the perfect you. You're forgiving of your shortcomings. Carrying a few extra pounds or having some wrinkles may affect how you look, but not *who you are*. When you respect yourself, you insist on being treated well by others.

Humanistic psychology, a field founded by Dr. Abraham Maslow, describes people with strong self-esteem as "self-actualized" human beings, people who have learned how to be as fully themselves as possible. It's this quality of perfect ease and self-acceptance that makes them attractive to others. The "self-actualized" person is bursting with inner beauty.

Getting real is a lifelong process, and it starts with six key steps:

1. Broaden your definition of beauty
2. Become more internally directed
3. Look outside yourself for life's meaning
4. Don't be afraid to entertain guilt-free feelings of pride
5. Enjoy fashion and beauty without becoming a slave to trends
6. Stay current with information, with ideas, with people

Nothing on the list about nose shape, cellulite, or breast size, is there? Did you really need a psychiatrist or dermatologist to tell you that big breasts won't make you happy? What will make you happy is enjoying the sight of yourself in family photos, attracting stimulating relationship partners, and loving that lady you see in the mirror.

Inner beauty means self-actualization, the affirmative act of making the most of your abilities and transcending your limitations wherever you can. Every woman possesses nearly limitless potential to love, be loved, and bring compassion and healing to those around her. On your journey, strive to develop the salient qualities of self-actualization. Radiant inner beauty is a quality of life that has nothing to do with your material possessions or wealth. It is the inner quality of life that shines. It costs nothing, and It's worth everything.

There is no area of the loop where it's more important to break free of the shackles of innate beauty and evolve to a place where you can look at the entire you and say, "Yeah, I'm pretty great."

BEAUTY BUDDIES

Lori Symans and Sandy Goor, sisters

Real estate sales-and-marketing professional Lori Symans and her sister, boutique owner Sandy Goor, can't seem to agree on who is younger. Sandy is younger by the calendar but insists that her sister actually looks two and a half years her junior. Be that as it may, they readily agree that they love doing a wide range of beauty-related activities together.

"Whatever Sandy does, I do," Lori says. "She's my role model for all things beauty. She's my idol as it relates to working out and staying in shape. She got a trainer; I got the same trainer. She does Botox; I do Botox. She owns a clothing store, and she dresses me. We do everything together."

The two ladies, who live in the Los Angeles area, use each other as beauty sounding boards—as all good girlfriends do. "We push each other and bounce ideas off of each other about different beauty products, regimens, where you got your latest haircut," says Sandy.

"A huge part of it is the rush, too," Lori says. "I recently lost twenty pounds, and we talk about how great it feels to be healthier. We get a rush out of feeling good and knowing that the things we do are natural. We like to have the rush of feeling beautiful from the inside, of living a good life and being good people."

Asked what each finds beautiful in the other, both ladies got a little emotional. "Lori is the best listener, with an open, kind heart," says Sandy. "She gives good feedback, but she knows it's more important to be that listening ear with an open heart."

As for Lori: "Sandy is the epitome of the person who puts her own issues aside and is there in the moment when she has to be there for you. She's the port in a storm who finds the positive in things for other people."

IF WE KNOW WHAT TO DO, WHY DON'T WE DO IT?

A big reason we've put self-esteem on such a high pedestal in this book is that poor self-esteem makes you unlikely to undertake significant changes in your life. Women with healthy self-esteem tend to believe that they can make lasting changes and that they deserve to be happier, so they act. Women with poor self-esteem often have defeatist attitudes that become disempowering internal narratives, such as "I never stick with anything; why even try?" Bringing about meaningful change always starts with loving yourself enough to try and knowing you can succeed.

Do you fall into the "I'll get to it one of these days" camp? Don't smile behind your hand! You know that some days you do. We all do. You know you need to eat right, work out, and wear sunscreen, but something stops you. That something is flawed inner beauty. Instead of working on what's inside, you're staring at those thirty extra pounds or those bags under your eyes and feeling helpless. You're starting in the wrong place. When you revitalize your self-esteem, inertia drops away naturally. Taking action becomes second nature, because you know you can be successful. So, let's start on the inside and work our way out.

ARE YOU SNOW WHITE OR THE WICKED QUEEN?

Having inner beauty means possessing women's finest qualities—kindness, self-love, passion, honor, empathy, humor, optimism, concern for the welfare of others, and confidence—in abundance and sharing them with the world. A woman who exhibits complete inner beauty does not let idle opinion influence her actions.

She knows that she's worth loving, and she loves who and what she is. If society thinks that she should have cosmetic surgery to erase those well-earned wrinkles, or that a woman her age should not be doing live poetry readings or protest marches . . . well, that's society's problem.

This is not arrogance. A woman with total inner beauty cares what others think of her actions. She wants to be regarded as honest, compassionate, and generous. She doesn't see herself as superior to other people. It's just that within her shines an unimpeachable core of knowledge that she is the best she can be. The opinion that carries the most weight is her own.

She knows that it's who you are, not what you look like, that makes you beautiful. To illustrate, let's use the example of Snow White and her stepmother, the wicked queen. The queen was beautiful but unspeakably vain, so much so that she couldn't stand the idea of there being any woman in the world more beautiful than she was. When told that Snow White exceeded her in beauty, she plotted to have her killed.

Because of her insecurity and envy, this physically attractive woman became emotionally and spiritually ugly. Her inability to accept herself without comparison with other women manifested itself in her anger, contorted expressions, and destructive actions. No prince would have any interest in the wicked queen. Contrast this characterization with Snow White, who was truly beautiful because of her kindness, good humor, and caring nature in looking after the seven dwarves, who were, by all accounts, slobs. Had she not been physically attractive, Snow White would still have been a beautiful person who attracted suitors and whom people loved—though perhaps this would not have made for a memorable fairy tale.

What Do You Have When You "Have It All"?

The queen is reminiscent of today's modern woman, constantly comparing herself with other women and judging herself wanting. We burden ourselves with expectations: have a career, raise a family, contribute to the community, take care of our bodies. It's easy to let life get out of balance and feel guilty that we're not keeping up with the ideal woman who, so we've heard, is "having it all." No one has it all. If a woman lacks self-esteem, she can feel like a failure for not being perfect in every role. Worse, she feels that she's got to take on even more to prove herself.

Numerous books, talk-radio programs, and TV forums debate the question "Should women try to have it all?" For men, it's a nonissue. On this point, Gloria Steinem noted, "When I go around and speak on campuses, I still don't get young men standing up and saying, 'How can I combine career and family?'" According to a 2007 survey by the Pew Research Center, 60 percent of full-time working mothers would rather be working part-time, a 25 percent increase since 1997. Yet only one in four working mothers does work part-time. It seems we're holding ourselves to an unreachable standard, taking on more in the workplace yet still not giving ourselves permission to do less at home.

We speak from personal experience here. We're both mothers. Some days, it seems as if we have the best of both worlds, while on others, it just seems as if there isn't enough of us to go around.

That yearning leads some women to become what psychologist Eugene Sagan called a "pathological critic." We let our inner critical voice become vicious and drown out any positive self-talk. We blame ourselves when things go wrong. We unfavorably compare ourselves with others. Our inner voice becomes a personal terrorist who's on duty twenty-four hours a day, setting unreachable standards for us and berating us when we fail to reach them.

BEAUTY STORY: "JANINE"

Twenty-four-year-old dancer Janine came to see Eva because of depression and anxiety. She had been injured for the first time in her career and had stopped training. After a few sessions, Eva determined that Janine's inner critic had her feeling as if the injury was the end of her career. Her mood was also suffering because she was no longer getting the feel-good chemicals that come with regular workouts. After several sessions focused on developing a more realistic assessment of the current situation, Janine felt much better. Eva helped her find a professional trainer experienced in working with athletes and dancers. The trainer helped Janine come up with an exercise program in which she could do intense workouts without risking reinjury. She also saw Debra about some minor cosmetic touch-ups.

Debra: *I was surprised when Janine came to see me. Here was this young woman in the kind of incredible condition you see only in professional dancers and athletes, and yet she was terribly anxious about her fitness level.*

Eva: *She is in a profession in which body shape and weight are extremely sensitive issues. Dancers feel intense pressure to keep themselves thin and graceful, because if you fall short of the high standards, there's some other dancer waiting to take your place.*

Debra: *When you helped her reinvent her workout, she got that sense of control back.*

This negative inner voice doesn't allow us to forgive ourselves for not living up to the myth of the "modern woman" who can work fourteen hours, bring home a big paycheck, breeze into the house after a long day looking fabulous, whip up a gourmet meal without leaving a measuring spoon out of place, read a bedtime story (which she wrote in her spare time) to the kids, and be a responsive lover to her lucky husband.

Trying to emulate that impossible model is highly stressful. Women with strong self-esteem don't try. They don't need to "have it all" in the clichéd sense, so they can forgive themselves for not being perfect and can celebrate what they already do well. They have *metacognition*, the ability to step back from their own thought process, and can catch themselves in self-defeating thinking. They're able to recognize how they respond to life and develop a healthy outlook, so they don't try to carry around all the "buckets" of life—work, family, volunteering—at once. When your self-esteem is strong, you don't need to be all things to all people in order to feel valuable. There's no impulse to beat yourself up for what you can't do. You do what you can do in the best, most giving way possible, and your value emanates from within.

No matter what you do, work at accurate self-assessment. Get to know your strengths, and take pride in them. Get to know your weaknesses, and make a plan to improve on them. Learn to describe yourself *to yourself* in a positive way. Give yourself a break once in a while. You'll defang your worst critic—you—and begin to think of yourself differently. That's magic that others will see.

LIVING INSIDE OUT

Every stage of the Beauty-Brain Loop affects the other three, and none packs more wallop than inner beauty. We'll state it as plainly as possible:

Your outward appearance, the environment you create,
and the environment's response to you are all reflections
of what's going on in your inner self.

Your evolving beauty, which grants you the ability to control how you see yourself and how others see you, hinges on
your mental and emotional health. When we say that habitual
thought patterns of anger, dependency, or self-loathing are toxic,
we're not being dramatic: they're like caustic chemicals dumped
into the rivers of your relationships. Because those relationships
all flow from you, if you poison the waters, everything starts
to die—but if the waters are pristine and healthy, downstream
relationships flourish and can even thrive through hard times.
You create your environment, and only you can make it truly
beautiful.

Your inner beauty affects the other stages of the loop in a
wide variety of ways:

• **Self-care:** This is one of the most basic ways in which inner
beauty shapes outer beauty. If you love yourself and feel that
you deserve to look your best, you take good care of yourself.
You work out, eat right, don't smoke, get enough sleep, care for
your skin, and do all the other things that bring about radiant
health and maximize your innate gifts. If you feel hopeless or
self-critical, you probably let your body go.

• **Facial appearance:** Negative emotions can alter the appearance of the face by triggering stress hormones that cause acne
outbreaks; dilating the pupils, which makes eye color appear to
change; and bringing on frowns and scowls that can etch lasting
lines. Some mind-body theorists even speculate that emotions can
actually bring about physical changes in the face on their own.

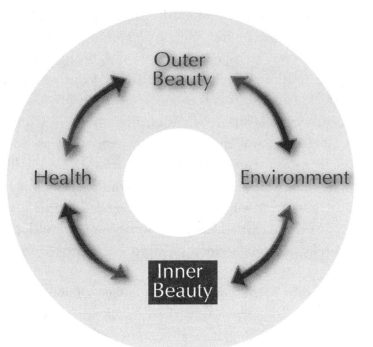

- **Social status:** Your standing in your social circle has less to do with how you look than with your personality type. Studies have shown that in a dormitory situation, women with extroverted personalities enjoyed higher social standing among both sexes than women who tended to be neurotic or withdrawn, no matter how physically attractive or unattractive the women were.

- **Grooming:** When you are convinced that you're average and no one will ever love you because of it, do you really think you are going to spend money on stylish clothing or that you'll get your hair done regularly? You take care of yourself only if you think you're worth the effort.

• **Managing stress:** Stressful events can be interpreted in constructive ways. For example: "Here is the problem; it's up to me to find the best way to cope with it. I need to breathe and figure out what to do next." This positive self-talk helps you develop ways to shield yourself from the damaging effects of stress. Practicing regular stress busters, such as meditation or yoga, prepares you to handle stressful situations while remaining as calm as possible. If instead, you interpret every stressor in your life as being something you deserved or can't handle, then your body will constantly be in the fight-or-flight mode. Negative inner beauty may even make you feel as if you *deserve* the health effects of stress: migraines, high blood pressure, or a wrecked immune system.

• **Relationships:** How you think of yourself can outweigh even strong physical attractiveness in the eyes of others. When you are hypercritical or embarrassed about yourself, you set off alarm bells in others, warning them that you are a drama queen, a burden, or just depressing to be around. Turn on the confidence and charm, and you send your attractiveness through the roof.

• **Overall health:** Bad moods can do real harm to your health. Chronic depression can lead to headaches, backaches, muscle pain, poor sleep, and possibly even decreased immune functioning and cardiovascular damage. A 2007 World Health Organization study published in *Lancet*, encompassing more than 245,000 people in sixty countries, showed that depression has a greater negative impact on health than angina, arthritis, asthma, and diabetes and is in fact a leading cause of disability worldwide.

The loop is *accelerative*. When you start doing things that change your inner beauty, that change picks up speed like a car rolling down a hill. Adopt positive attitudes and start exercising,

---

BEAUTY PEARLS

If you feel beautiful within yourself and have a beautiful heart and soul, your beauty will shine within and other people around you will feel it. Most important, you will feel it. I think in our society you should not worry about what color, size, or shape you are or where you might be from and realize you are beautiful and unique in your own way. Someone out there will recognize the beauty you have to share with others and the beauty that surrounds you."

—Lisa Pliner, fashion director, Donald J. Pliner of Florida, Inc.

---

and you find that as you feel better and better, you start dressing better, and your social life improves. Spend your nights accusing your reflection of being fat, and it's not long before you've surrendered all thoughts of being in shape. Once the car is rolling, it's hard to stop. Thousands of women turn their lives around every year, but it's easier to start by driving in the right direction in the first place.

THE BIG O

One aid to getting through difficult times with your inner beauty intact is optimism. The more you can train yourself to respond optimistically to what life sends your way, the stronger your self-esteem and the healthier your thought patterns will be. At the opposite end of the spectrum from distorted thinking are the kind of healthy, supportive mental habits that breed optimism. We call them "the Big O." That stands for *optimism*, not that other word.

The best habit is simply to start replacing negative thoughts with positive ones. Optimism can be learned, and you learn it the same way you learn anything else: through repetition. When you feel a negative thought coming on, turn it on its head by an act of will. Replace "I can't lose the weight" with "I will take steps today to start losing the weight." The present doesn't change (you still need to lose the weight), but your approach to tomorrow is completely different. Every day, we act as judge and jury of our own actions. Rule yourself innocent. Some self-criticism keeps you honest and motivates, but being overly self-critical can damage self-esteem.

Optimism also requires pride, and that's easiest when you're a good person. What does it mean to be a good person? To us, it means adopting a set of principles and living by them. It means having honor. It means giving your word and sticking to it. These are old-fashioned ideas, but that doesn't matter; they're timeless. When others know you will do what you say you'll do and act according to a set of rules that you never violate, they'll respect you, and you'll respect yourself.

Another part of the Big O is the idea of honoring yourself. We tend to "aw shucks" even our finest moments, but why should we? When you've acted with courage or done something that brings joy to another person, take a moment to bask in the glow. Acknowledge that you have behaved in a way that's worth being recognized. Don't share the feeling with anyone else; it could be misconstrued as conceit. Just enjoy a private time knowing you "done good." Learning to identify and appreciate times when you feel good will enhance your overall sense of well-being. Bask in the moment if you feel pride, joy, sexual excitement, or other wonderful sensations.

BEAUTY BOOSTERS

Practical things you can do now to be more beautiful

Consider your closest relationships. Being near a judgmental person who issues harsh criticisms zaps beauty. During this journey from "powerless" to "powerhouse," you may need to erect some firm boundaries or discontinue toxic relationships altogether. This move is difficult, because it requires you to alter habits that have built up over years and to change the rules of power with the people you know. Do it anyway. Stand up to a "friend" or family member who has made it a practice over the years to criticize your appearance or to make you feel unattractive. Do it calmly but firmly—not chastising the other person, but having the courage not to be kicked around anymore. Take control. You will be astonished at how good it makes you feel.

It's just as important to honor others. We can go off and sit in a cave and meditate for years, but we really find out what happened in that cave only when we come out and get involved with other people. Participate in life. Get out there and engage, and do it with people who are positive and hopeful about the world. You'll learn more about yourself and others in a weekend helping beauty professionals give makeovers to homeless women than in a year spent alone.

Finally, embrace your spiritual side. This doesn't mean simply running off to join a religious institution, but certainly, belonging to a group does give people a sense of community, especially at times of celebration and crisis. Plus, research has shown that people with deep religious or spiritual beliefs enjoy greater health and longevity. If you have a faith, invest in it. Find out what it means to you and if it really speaks to you. If you're unsure, make an effort to read, talk, and discover. Spirituality is about meaning, not doctrine. Seek out something that resonates with that something inside you that's not about achievement or logic: nature, music, meditation, philosophy. Let yourself ask the big questions. What are they? That's up to you.

LOOK BETTER, FEEL BETTER

Inner beauty is within your control. You just have to make the conscious decision to stop that car from rolling down the hill and turn it around. Emotions are habitual patterns of responding to the events and people in our lives. Those habits can be deeply ingrained into our brains, especially if they took root during childhood, but we can also change those patterns by taking conscious action. The brain is changeable.

To improve your self-talk and change negative patterns, it helps to improve your appearance. Numerous studies have indicated that people who had successful dental or cosmetic surgery to correct problems with their appearance experienced significantly improved self-esteem and quality of life.

You don't have to opt for cosmetic surgery. Start with your hair or skin, or simply get out and exercise. Fitness makes any woman look more attractive. Even better, try combining healthy exercise with an appreciation for the beauty around you by walking, running, cycling, or playing tennis or golf (remember your sunscreen). A Dutch study revealed that exercising outdoors in pleasing urban or rural scenery can lower blood pressure, improve self-esteem, and increase the enjoyment of exercise. In fact, even the color green is healthful; in a 2004 study at a college in the Southeast, the sight of the color green evoked feelings of relaxation, calmness, happiness, comfort, peace, hope, and excitement. If you can't get outside, go to the gym or aerobics studio. Exercising regularly and feeling yourself become fitter, stronger, and more flexible is a tonic for the self-image.

At the same time, avoid the things that sap your inner beauty. Addictive substances are your enemy. Whether it's nicotine or alcohol, addiction means you're not in control. Another pitfall is putting yourself into situations in which you know you're going to be overly critical of yourself, such as visiting a nightclub frequented by women twenty years younger than

---

BEAUTY BUSTERS

Beauty myths debunked while you wait

Myth: Attractive people have higher self-esteem.
Fact: Self-esteem is not a light switch to be flipped on, nor is it magically conferred by good looks. Researchers studying the effect of physical attractiveness on self-esteem surveyed a broad segment of the population for self-esteem and also obtained photos of each respondent. They then asked a panel to try to determine, based only on the photos, who had the highest self-esteem. In that study, self-reported physical attractiveness had a strong correlation with self-esteem, independent of objective opinions of the subjects' attractiveness. People with high-self esteem apparently find themselves beautiful, even if others do not.

Do people with high self-esteem take better care of themselves and therefore look better? Maybe. The relationship between self-esteem and beauty is like that between the chicken and the egg. In any case, the evidence says that if you have strong self-esteem, your evolved sense of your own beauty is also strong.

you. Being self-aware means putting yourself in a position to succeed rather than setting yourself up to brood.

PLAY TO YOUR STRENGTHS

You need to know your strengths, mental and physical, and emphasize them. Can you realistically appraise your strengths and weaknesses right now? That's the level of self-awareness you want. If a woman with great eyes can emphasize them with dramatic eye makeup, why can't you bring out your best inner feature? If you are smart and have a great sense of humor, become the witty spark for every social gathering. You won't be the best in every situation; if you try to be, you'll only wind up feeling inadequate. Just let your strength shine and let someone else have the spotlight. Not needing the spotlight to be on you all the time is a hallmark of healthy self-esteem.

What are your inner strengths? Are you cultivating them? Are you making the most you can of them? What weaknesses are you willing to live with? Is there a way to turn some of them into strengths? Asking these questions has one terrific instant side effect: you start to see your strengths more clearly. If you're not sure about your strong suits, ask a trusted friend for an honest opinion.

MENTAL TOOLS FOR DAILY LIVING

The female mind and emotions are subtle and complicated. So, there are just as many tools and ideas for improving inner beauty as there are types of women. Here are a few we really like:

• **Look for beauty around you.** Remember our bird-watching exercise? Training your eye to recognize beauty in settings that you might not have previously seen as beautiful can retrain your brain and stimulate new neural pathways. This keeps your brain young as you age and helps change unhealthy thought patterns.

- **Practice random kindness.** Do something considerate and unexpected for someone with no thought of reward.
- **Set achievable goals.** When we accomplish things, we feel good about ourselves. This is the source of genuine self-esteem. Don't set your goals so high that you can't reach them with a stepladder. Make them realistic enough so you can succeed and feel good about it. You can always set tougher goals later on when you've gained more confidence.
- **Bring humor into life.** Go to comedy clubs, read humorous books, or hang out with funny people. Life is funny if you can see the humor.
- **Give to others.** Volunteer. Donate. Help poor people. Bill Clinton had a bestseller in 2007 simply called *Giving* and launched an organization called My Commitment to encourage others to give and change the world. Oprah Winfrey donates generously to charity and supports causes such as starting girls' schools in Africa. They and millions of others know that making a difference in someone's life is a wonderful way to feel great about oneself.
- **Love and be loved.** Savor your relationships. Express your love for your family and friends every way you can, especially if you've been together a while.
- **Be affirmative.** Tell yourself what you want to be true, and say it out loud: "I am beautiful. I am smart. I am capable. I can figure this out. I deserve to be happy. I am a good person. Life is good." You will be amazed at how much power verbalizing those ideas has to alter your mood and your ability to cope.
- **Try new things.** Take some risks; stick your neck out a little. It feels exhilarating to master something you haven't tried before.

- **Express your creativity.** If you write, paint, or sing, go for it. If you don't do any of those things, you can still be creative. Redesign a room in your home. Arrange flowers. Develop a stimulating lesson for your children. Cook. The ways to express your creative passion are limitless.
- **Stimulate yourself intellectually.** Take a class, read a difficult book, see an opera in Italian, without subtitles. Challenge your mind.
- **Be flexible.** Things won't always go your way. When they don't, don't freak out. Adapt. Spontaneity is like hot sauce for living. Sometimes, the greatest ideas you'll ever have will come when your grand plans fall through.
- **Make sure your work is enhancing your inner beauty.** If your work life saps your spirit, can you try a new job? If you can't, find ways to do your job differently.
- **Be grateful.** Remember to be thankful for your family, your health, your home, and your life. Not everyone has these gifts.
- **Surround yourself with beautiful people.** Inner beauty is contagious.
- **Follow your passion.** You say you've always wanted to learn to play the piano? What's stopping you?

We saved passion for last because it's something women often neglect. We see women rushing around with their hair on fire, never taking time to do the things they love because of the things they "have to do." If you take a day off work to do something you love, not only will work wait for you, but also you'll be happier and work better when you get back to the office. Spending some of your time doing something you're passionate about is a prescription for energy, joy, and vitality. We have patients who've quit successful careers to go back to the full-time pursuit of passions such as photography or art, and guess what? They're still making livings, and their lives are far sweeter for the change. Others make time after work to indulge in a passion. These experiences create memories that last a lifetime and create real beauty in our hectic lives.

Beauty Bullets

- Inner beauty is all about self-esteem.

- "Having it all" is frequently a trap for women.

- Much of poor inner beauty derives from distorted thinking.

- Learn to be an optimist.

- Your inner beauty drives all other loop stages.

- Looking better is a tried-and-true way to feel better.

- Attitudes and emotions can be habits.

- Passion is a wonderful beauty elixir.

 BEAUTY AND THE BRAIN Rx

Knowing Yourself

Dr. Eva: *Read Dr. Martin Seligman's classic book* Learned Optimism. *In his research, Seligman found that optimistic people are happier than pessimists.*

(continued)

When something bad happens, optimists think of it as temporary, limited in its effect, and not their fault. Pessimists consider the setback to be permanent, far-reaching, and all their fault. Researchers report that optimism contributes to good health and greater life success, while pessimism contributes to illness and more frequent failure.

Optimism and pessimism both tend to be self-fulfilling prophecies. If you think a setback is permanent, you won't try to change the conditions that led to it. Optimistic explanations make you more likely to act. If you think the setback is temporary, you're apt to try to do something about it, and because you take action, you make it temporary. As Henry Ford said, "Whether you think that you can, or that you can't, you are usually right."

Dr. Debra: *Women are natural caretakers and sometimes neglect to take care of themselves. Remember to take care of yourself the way you take care of others. Make sure you are allotting time each day to nurture your own health and beauty. Make a standing appointment with yourself for at least ten minutes twice a day: schedule "beauty time" to perform self-care or just relax.*

5

Health: The Five Cards of Lifelong Wellness

A woman's health is her capital.

— Harriet Beecher Stowe

I T'S A FABULOUS house, the kind most of us wish we owned. Maybe it's a villa on the Amalfi Coast of Italy or a modern-day palace in Beverly Hills. It's magnificent, classy, stunning. It's appointed with fine artwork, Italian marble, a kitchen to die for, hand-painted frescoes, and a rose garden worthy of Versailles. It's a showplace that's been featured in *Architectural Digest*. There's just one thing wrong: this grand house is crumbling. Unseen by anyone, its foundation is cracked and slowly subsiding into the earth below it. The wiring is outdated. The wood frame is ridden with termites. This splendid edifice is ready to topple over in the next strong storm—or, if it's in Beverly Hills, the next big earthquake.

When it comes to beauty, your foundation is what you have to work with even if you don't have a dime to spend on makeup or nice clothes. It's fitness, diet, sleep, hydration, and all the other behaviors that help determine how healthy you are. The things you must go out and get—power suits, a trendy haircut, cosmetic surgery—are decoration, furnishings for your body and mind. It's wonderful to have beautiful furnishings, like the house with the travertine and Sub-Zero appliances, but the furnishings don't matter much if your foundation is falling apart. You can spend a fortune on world-class cosmetics and have the finest fashion designers in Paris on speed dial, but you'll still look unattractive if your eyes have bags big enough to have "Prada" embroidered on them.

WHEN "SIX-PACK" DOESN'T MEAN BEER

The foundation of beauty is health of body. If you're not healthy, it's difficult to be physically attractive, and it's nearly impossible to have that personal magnetism that stops people in their tracks. For most of us, true attractiveness comes in part from radiating health that others can sense and see. That's our tricky DNA at work again.

People unconsciously look for signs of health in others, because their health suggests their fitness as a mate. A man's six-pack abs and bulging biceps get women's attention (in part) because a thousand magazine covers and reruns of "Baywatch" have convinced us that they're sexy, but go deeper and you find that innate sense of beauty again, that programmed physical ideal. From the perspective of genetically inherited innate beauty, rippling muscles mean a man is fit enough to live many years and father many children, powerful enough to hunt and provide for his family, and swift enough to fight off marauding tribes. Let's see David Hasselhoff do that.

Biology is also behind the female need to primp, perfume, and make ourselves more attractive. As Yvonne Antelle wrote in *How to Catch and Hold a Man* (and Maureen Dowd quoted memorably in the *New York Times*), "Keep thinking of yourself as a soft, mysterious cat. . . . Men are fascinated by bright, shiny objects, by lots of curls, lots of hair on the head . . . by bows, ribbons, ruffles, and bright colors. . . . Sarcasm is dangerous. Avoid it altogether." Fair or not, we want to dazzle romantic partners so we will be chosen. We all want to look our best, and that simply must begin with optimal health.

There is a downside to this female genetic predisposition to make ourselves look alluring, however: it encourages shortcuts. We wear shiny earrings, have our hair professionally styled, and

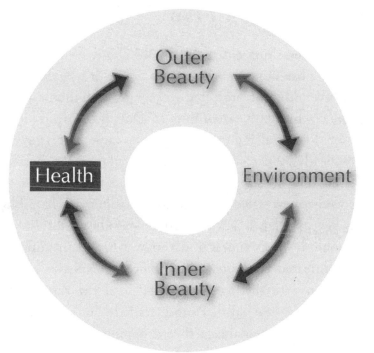

slink into a little black dress right out of an Audrey Hepburn movie, but we overlook the importance of cutting back on our saturated fats and not smoking. A well-dressed, slender exterior can hide truly poor health (at least temporarily) if people aren't looking too closely. It's easy to get lazy.

For your sake, don't take the shortcuts. Look as stylish and put together as possible, but start with a vigorous foundation of physical wellness. For us or any other physicians, the true goal is to keep our patients well, rather than treating them after they become sick. We would rather see you begin your journey to real, magnetic beauty by making a long-term investment in your health. Not only will it help you lead a longer, fuller life, but also it will enhance all the other stages of the Beauty-Brain Loop.

SCALES ARE FOR FISH

Let us make one thing clear: this is not about weight. Weight is a national obsession, especially for women. If it weren't, U.S. consumers wouldn't be projected to spend $54 billion a year on diet products by 2009, according to Datamonitor. It doesn't seem to be doing much good, though: the same report says that by 2009, nearly 70 percent of the U.S. population is expected to be overweight or obese.

For women, excessive concern about weight can be a blight on life. The problem is not limited to serious eating disorders such as bulimia and anorexia nervosa, which can ruin your health or threaten your life. It also encompasses the constant preoccupation with dieting and weight loss, the thousands of dollars spent in a year on diet products that don't deliver what they promise, and the damage that dropping a few pounds via a radical diet and then putting it back on inflicts on a woman's body. Researchers have learned that excessive yo-yo dieting

BEAUTY BUDDIES

Linda Leibovitch and Tracey Hampton-Stein

Linda and Tracey are more than Beauty Buddies; they have a shared commitment to political activism that mirrors their commitment to activities that make them feel more beautiful.

"Tracey is inspiring to me because she is a success in her own right, and as an African-American woman, she has faced more challenges than most," says Linda. The two women began sharing time when they worked on their first political fund-raiser together and became fast friends. They have built a relationship around "being there" for each other through campaigns, health problems, the needs of kids, or everyday crises of all kinds. With Tracey spending half the year in Florida while Linda is based in Southern California, the two spend a great deal of their time on the phone but get together for Starbucks or sushi whenever and wherever they can.

"The experience of having Tracey as a friend has changed my life," says Linda. "Because of her, I found my passion and the courage to pursue it. I don't think that was possible in my thirties. Watching her maneuver in the world is so inspirational. She will use her substantial influence in the political world only to help someone else. She is a role model who has taught me how to be elegant while interacting with the world."

The greatest lesson Linda has learned from her Beauty Buddy relationship? "Don't be afraid to reach out," she says. "It feels good to be able to help another person, and feeling good inside is what ultimately makes us beautiful on the outside."

causes restriction of blood flow to the heart as well as a compromised immune system.

Obesity is a serious risk factor for disease and should always be dealt with. However, in a quest for a quick fix for being overweight, some women are harming their health and ignoring the psychological issues that sometimes underlie poor habits. So, we'll state it clearly: there are no shortcuts. Most diet programs and products don't work in the long term. They are a temporary solution to a permanent need. Some are downright unhealthy. To lose weight, increase the number of calories you burn, and reduce the calories you take in. Granted, this takes a committed lifestyle change, and that can seem impossible when you're doing your superwoman impression from dawn to midnight.

We suggest this: don't make your weight your gauge of beauty. Throw away your scale. Most personal trainers will tell you not to worry about the scale anyway, but to focus on how your clothes fit. Instead of fixating on pounds and inches, set your sights on getting and staying healthy.

Here's a news flash you may not have seen in the mainstream media: **You don't necessarily have to be slim to be healthy.** Blasphemy, right? It is in a world where size-zero models are celebrated and every magazine in the checkout line is bursting with headlines about miracle diets that will help you lose twenty pounds in thirty days (extremely unlikely and probably dangerous). We're brainwashed to believe that unless we can bounce a quarter off our glutes, we're out of shape and ugly.

MAKE THE MOST OF WHAT YOU'RE GIVEN

It's certainly preferable to be as close to your ideal weight as possible. However, you can be in ideal cardiovascular shape, strong from strength training or Pilates, and fortified by eating a terrific diet filled with fruits, vegetables, nuts, and lean protein—and still be thick in the waist or wide in the hips. We see it all the time, especially in women over fifty whose metabolisms have downshifted. Maybe your body type means you'll never be waif-thin. Perhaps your natural metabolic rate tells your body to store extra fat, and you can't lose it no matter how hard you work.

So what? Your body is the hand of cards you're dealt by your genetic heritage, and that's something in which you don't have any say. That doesn't mean you have to fold. You can play smart and improve your cards. A lot.

We know women whose bodies are hardly perfect, but hook them up to a cardiac stress-test machine and they're ready to run a 10K. They work out regularly and eat well, and they're fit because of it. Know what? They're *happy*. They're magnetic. They feel like a million bucks, and it's obvious. Exercise is a great mood booster, but that's not the only reason they're so giddy. They have megawatts of energy and the peace of mind that comes with knowing they're taking care of themselves. They know they've made the most of the hand of cards that their DNA dealt them.

That's what we advise you to do. Forget about weight. Think fit. Think healthy. Think strong and flexible and lean and energetic. Bring out the absolute peak of what your genetics will allow by committing to healthful habits and you'll feel the way those ladies do. And if you happen to end up with a body that has people on the street mistaking you for an aerobics teacher, that's a bonus.

FIVE OF A KIND

What we're talking about here is *wellness*, being not just healthy but also filled with pride and optimism because you know you're doing everything to ensure that you live long, well, and wonderfully. Part of the glow of wellness comes from being in control of how you look. You're not just taking whatever cards nature slides across the green felt of life, sighing, and saying with resignation, "I'll play these." You're taking command of the game. You're betting on yourself and raising the stakes. You're deciding what your body is capable of. That's evolving beauty at its finest.

The components of true wellness make up a perfect five-card poker hand—a royal flush, in fact. Knowing how to play those cards to your advantage does more than help you optimize your inborn physical gifts. It gives you something many women never enjoy: the freedom to defy many of the stereotypes of aging. No matter how old you are now, that's a real gift.

The five cards of lasting health and wellness are these:

1. Exercise
2. Nutrition
3. Sleep
4. Stress management
5. Health care

How to play them depends on who you are and how you've lived your life so far. If you've got questions about how to work out or what to eat, talk to a personal trainer or a dietitian. We're neither, but we can definitely get you moving in the right direction. We're not going to spend a lot of time rehashing the advice you can get from a hundred other books and magazine articles. We'll hit the essentials but give the information a bit of *The Beauty Prescription* panache. Let's deal the cards.

The Ace: Exercise

If you're a woman looking for the elixir of long life, exercise is your drinking fountain. Exercise has so many restorative qualities and benefits that if you can play only one card in the wellness game, make it the ace. Exercise hard and regularly, and have fun doing it.

The more you move, the healthier you'll be. The less you move, the greater your risk of disease. We interviewed Kathy Kaehler, a celebrity personal trainer, a regular on the "Today Show," and author of *Fit and Sexy for Life*, and she told us, "You need a routine on a day-to-day basis that engages your muscles and elevates your heart rate. People think, 'I can't imagine doing an aerobics class or going out running.' You don't have to do those things. You can take a walk after dinner or take a bike ride around your neighborhood. You have to make exercise a lifestyle."

A BRIEF (MENO)PAUSE. Even if you're in your twenties (and if you are, good for you for reading this book), one of these days you'll hit the life transition called menopause. You may already be there or beyond. In any case, it's a time when changes hit your body like a runaway freight train. Your metabolic rate can slow, and you start to gain weight around your middle. You lose bone density, increasing your risk of osteoporosis and fractures. Sex can become uncomfortable. Your self-esteem takes a hit. And here's worse news: your risk of heart disease goes up. That's right. After age sixty, more women die from heart disease than men. Before menopause, your hormones protected you, but after? Sorry, you're on your own.

Some women cruise through menopause, while others have a rough ride, with hot flashes, unpredictable emotions, and other symptoms. No matter who you are or how old you are, changes come with age, and the smartest way to weather them is to take positive action and get yourself as fit as possible. As Kaehler writes in her book, "There isn't one side effect of meno-

---

BEAUTY STORY: "SANDRA"

This twenty-nine-year-old woman, who'd given birth six weeks before, went to see Debra about her stretch marks. She was tearful and depressed far out of proportion to her skin condition, so Debra referred her to a psychiatrist while prescribing topical creams to prevent worsening of the stretch marks.

Eva: Depression after giving birth is remarkably common. Studies have shown that it can strike one woman in seven. In this discussion, it's important to distinguish the "baby blues" from true depression. Baby blues occur in most women after giving birth but usually go away within a couple of weeks, whereas postpartum depression is a serious illness requiring medical attention.

Debra: I see a lot of baby blues, because some women are unhappy with their bodies after giving birth. They might have gained too much weight, be experiencing skin changes or hair loss, or have unrealistic expectations for how fast their body will bounce back.

Eva: You can't set your expectations based on other women's experiences. No matter how your body responds to pregnancy, if you eat well, exercise, and maintain a healthy weight, you're going to bounce back faster.

---

pause—from mood swings to lack of energy—that exercise can't improve!"

Regardless of your age, there are four types of exercise you should consider incorporating into your life:

1. Aerobic. Examples include running, cycling, swimming, tennis, aerobics classes, stair climbing, and elliptical machines. You should do at least thirty minutes of aerobic exercise at least five days a week.

2. Strength training. Muscle burns twenty times more calories than fat does, so the more lean muscular weight you have on your body, the more calories you'll burn in daily activity. In addition, weight-bearing exercise helps you grow new bone mass, preventing osteoporosis, which makes so many older women vulnerable to broken bones. You should lift weights two to three times per week, targeting different muscle groups.

3. Flexibility. Stretching, yoga, and Pilates promote flexibility. Yoga or Pilates two days a week is fine, but you should be stretching after each workout when your muscles are supple. Aim for ten to fifteen minutes of steady stretching (no lunging, which can cause muscle injury).

4. Balance. As you get older, balance is especially important to prevent falls. The National Institutes of Health's recommendation is to incorporate balance exercises into your strength-training routine. One good way is to do leg raises two to three times a week in between your weight lifting.

THROW YOURSELF A CURVE . . . OR GO TO BED. Hate gyms? You're not alone. *The Beauty Prescription* take on exercise is to vary it and make it fun. There are dozens of ways to get your heart pumping, and most of them get you out of the gym. Try dancing or tennis. Go for a long hike. We know a woman in her sixties named Emily who recently discovered Argentinian tango dancing and has become addicted to it—but in a positive way. The chemicals we secrete when we exercise are similar to opiates, which is why regular strenuous exercise is addicting. That's the one addiction we wholeheartedly endorse. Every time Emily goes out dancing, she gets an incredible workout and has a fantastic time doing it. Last we spoke, her main complaint was that she was being picked up by men thirty years her junior! Go, girl.

You should also surprise your body by varying your workout. Do a longer workout on the weekends, for example. Varying your program helps you avoid those infamous, maddening plateaus, when your body becomes accustomed to the demands of a certain exercise routine, and weight loss slows or stops. Also, take advantage of the fact that we women are social creatures by making your workout a communal experience. Take a yoga class, hire a trainer, or enlist workout partners. You'll enjoy the motivation and the companionship.

And let's not forget about sex. It's a marvelous workout. It burns about one hundred calories an hour and can be a lot more fun than a treadmill. "You'll strengthen your quads, hamstrings, and abs and burn calories," says Laura Berman, Ph.D., author of *The Passion Prescription: Ten Weeks to Your Best Sex—Ever!* As long as you have safe sex, getting close with your partner has numerous health benefits, including being seen as beautiful and seeing your partner as beautiful. And few things defuse a stressful day better.

No time to exercise, you say? Sorry, that dodge doesn't fly here. Kaehler teaches her clients simple five-minute workouts that get your heart pumping and your body sweating. "Everyone can spare five minutes," she points out. "I teach a whole series of five-minute routines: jumping jacks, which provide impact that's good for the bones; sitting against the wall, which engages the lower body; forward lunges, a lower-body strengthener; military push-ups; bicycle crunches. You can do each one in five minutes, and by the end of your day, you've gotten a workout."

EXERCISE SMART. Remember to use your brain when you exercise. In other words, be smart and safe about it. There is a risk of injury with any exercise, so embark on a workout program that's safe for your body. Check with your doctor or a certified athletic trainer or physical therapist to make sure you can handle the exercise regimen to which you aspire.

If you go cycling, wear a helmet. If you're exercising outdoors, always wear sunscreen. If you're in a class such as spinning or aerobics, make sure your instructor is certified, and don't risk injuring yourself in trying to keep up with the other students. Listen to your body, and remember that some sports, such as martial arts or rock climbing, carry an inherently higher risk of injury.

As we get older, it becomes all the more important to exercise carefully. Our muscles are not as supple as they used to be, and it can be imperative to warm up by walking or stretching before a workout. Most trainers advise a short warm-up session before a workout, as well as a cooldown period afterward, plus stretching while your muscles are warm and flexible. Eat light, complex carbohydrates before a workout so you'll have energy without feeling sluggish, and follow your workout by eating protein, which boosts metabolism and helps muscles rebuild.

Start at a pace that works for you, and remember that maintaining your fitness program is the passport to success.

The King: Nutrition

The other top card in our health hand is all about what you put in your body: not just food, but also water and supplements. You should be eating mostly fresh, unprocessed food: fruit, vegetables, nuts, seeds, whole grains. This kind of eating ensures that you'll consume a healthful dose of just about the best wellness tonic there is: antioxidants and phytonutrients. Antioxidants, including vitamins E and C, selenium, and zinc, fight the cellular damage that occurs as a side effect of turning food into fuel. Phytonutrients, which appear in whole foods from vanilla beans to tea leaves, are chemicals that are not fully understood, nor is it known how many there are yet. We do know that they impart health-enhancing and disease-preventing benefits. Phytonutrients are one big reason that foods such as red grapes, green tea, and walnuts help prevent cancer and heart disease.

The full value lies in eating the whole food. For example, so far as science can tell, the greatest benefit of broccoli comes from eating the entire stalk, possibly because the fiber serves as a delivery system, or because of other compounds we don't yet know exist. This means no cheating by eating junk and then taking supplements to make up for dietary sins. "Although supplements may have some benefit, I do not always use them in my nutritional plans," says Katherine McCune, a registered dietitian and medical nutrition therapist. "There has been some controversy about supplements and possible toxicity levels. So many foods now are fortified with nutrients—calcium in orange juice, energy bars, and so on—that consumers are ingesting large amounts of nutrients along with supplements. Now people have to be careful about not oversupplementing.

"A lot of people think supplements will compensate for a bad diet," McCune continues, "but there are so many micronutrients we don't even know about in fresh food that you have to start there."

McCune runs down her top ten list of the best beauty-brain foods women should be consuming regularly. Ideally, these foods should be unprocessed and free of preservatives and pesticides. These foods, used in a daily meal plan of three meals and one to two snacks, contribute to a healthful variety of carbohydrates, protein and fat, vitamins, and minerals:

- Plenty of water to plump the skin and stay well hydrated
- Berries—any variety from blueberries to strawberries and beyond; all berries are antioxidant powerhouses
- Tropical fruits such as guava, kiwifruit, and pineapple
- Foods rich in omega-3 and omega-6 fatty acids: avocados, wild salmon, herring, mackerel, eggs, walnuts, canola oil, and soybeans
- All kinds of seeds and nuts, preferably unsalted
- Whole grains (the words *whole grain*—not just *whole wheat*—should appear on the ingredients label)
- Quality carbohydrates paired with good proteins (for example: ten almonds with a nectarine, or peanut butter on sesame crackers); this gives you a feeling of satiety (fullness) that you need, especially in the middle of the day, and keeps you from snacking on junk
- Selenium-rich foods such as tuna, whole wheat bread, and Brazil nuts
- High-fiber foods from whole grains to fresh vegetables

EATING AND YOUR BRAIN. Eating frequent, small meals can help in losing weight. If you deprive yourself of food, your body sends out more hunger signals and will do its best to make sure you pack on the calories when they become available. The reason is that our brains are designed to deal with a scarcity of food. Starvation was a real problem in the days when our brains were rapidly evolving. We are further programmed to love sweets and fats, because these were what kept our ancestors alive. We needed that positive response as motivation to remember where we found those tasty morsels. Probably nothing got us salivating like the sight of our men returning from the hunt with a big catch.

Today, our recalcitrant brains are having a hard time adapting to all this food we have around. It's easy to eat too much. Small, healthful snacks are satisfying, and we will have to wait for our brains to evolve to recognize that obesity, not starvation, is the real threat. In the meantime, we need to outsmart our urges, so don't think you can lose weight by going hungry. Your brain is too smart for that. Go ahead and eat; just make good, healthy choices.

TAKE JOY IN FOOD. Healthy eating is *attentive* eating, paying attention to all your food choices and not munching away on autopilot. If you're a typically busy, multitasking woman, you need to set yourself up for dietary success. Stock the kitchen with healthful snacks. Make sure the fresh ingredients you need for healthful meals are all available so you don't have to go shopping at the end of a long day, which can tempt you to eat packaged, unwholesome stuff.

Have a file of quick, light recipes at your fingertips. (A list of our favorite recipe and cooking websites is included in the Resources.) Our best advice is to learn to enjoy simple, fresh foods that require little or no preparation. Eat consciously, always aware of what you put into your body, and it becomes second nature to make good choices.

As with exercise, eating for wellness and beauty becomes a lifestyle. You learn to enjoy how really eating well makes you feel. If you don't cook much, test the waters with something basic. Preparing a yummy meal from fresh ingredients is a healthful,

BEAUTY BOOSTERS

Practical things you can do now to be more beautiful

Give yourself a "mind makeover." Just as it's healthy to change your appearance sometimes, you should also change your mental processes on occasion. Challenge yourself to see things in a different light. Spend time talking to someone with a different perspective, such as a person from a different age-group or background. Read an unfamiliar genre of book, or listen to a new type of music. Learn a new language. Make friends who are outside your usual experience. The process can be eye opening and invigorating for your brain.

healing experience and gives you control over what's on your plate; at a restaurant, you often have no idea how much fat or sodium you're swallowing. Also, get the freshest food you can find. At the market, troll the perimeter, where the produce, dairy, and fresh meats are arrayed. Shop at farmer's markets or, if you can, grow your own fruits, vegetables, and herbs. There's not much more satisfying than biting into a peppery tomato fresh from your backyard vine.

Above all, take a tip from the Europeans and make food a sensual experience, not just a refueling stop. Take time with your meals. Try to eat locally grown food when you can, for the experience of knowing where your food comes from. Eat slowly and from a full palette of foods. Savor what you eat and drink. Make dining a communal experience. Evoke the dinner scene from *A Year in Provence*: tables surrounded by friends, an assortment of foods fresh from the earth, meals that last for hours. You'll be more satisfied with your dining life, and you won't stand for anything but the best, healthiest food. Your beauty deserves nothing less.

The Queen: Sleep

If you're yawning during this game of cards, it's probably because you're denying your body what it wants: sleep. Shakespeare wrote that sleep "knits up the ravell'd sleeve of care" and that it is "chief nourisher in life's feast." We're guessing that if you've been playing the part of the career woman or full-time mom who tries to be all things to all people, you've been doing precious little knitting. Have we got a wake-up call for you.

A poll by the National Sleep Foundation showed that 22 percent of Americans are getting less sleep than they think they need, a deficit that leads to everything from poor work performance to loss of interest in sex. Not getting enough sleep also makes your body more likely to be "on alert" and producing stress hormones, so when true stress comes along, you're less able to handle it. And when you're tired all the time, you don't want to work out and probably don't care what you eat. Not getting enough sleep can be murder on your beauty habits.

"I'll sleep when I'm dead," smart alecks say. Some of us even regard our sleep deprivation with pride, as if working thirty hours without a break qualifies us for some sort of medal in the career Olympics. That's crazy. Medicine may not fully understand why our bodies sleep, but we know this: sleep is mandatory, and no amount of caffeine or other chemical can substitute.

For most women, six to eight hours of sleep is ideal. Men on average need an hour less, so don't fret if your husband or partner is a shorter sleeper than you. When you're in deep sleep, your body rests, ridding itself of the lactic acid that builds up when you work your muscles. Your immune system recharges. Your brain rests. If you doubt the power sleep has over your quality of life, start going to sleep an hour earlier each night and see how much better you feel.

Here's our sleep prescription:

- Create a sleep-friendly environment in your home. Customize your sleep space with pillows, fabrics, music—whatever you need to feel restful. Skip the candles; they're one of the most common causes of house fires. Substitute soft electric lanterns.
- Start a bedtime ritual. This can include bathing, meditation, yoga, reading, stargazing, or anything else that gets you in a relaxed state of mind.
- Avoid caffeine six hours before bedtime.
- Avoid alcohol or exercise two hours before bedtime. Although alcohol may put you to sleep, it prevents you from reaching the restorative phases of sleep, so you wake feeling poorly rested.
- If you need to relax, try caffeine-free herbal teas such as valerian or chamomile. Even the act of sipping warm tea can be overpoweringly restful.
- Go to bed at the same time as often as you can. This helps "set" your body's internal clock so that you become tired as this time gets closer. Waking up at the same time every morning will also help.
- Block out all external light and sound. Your sleep chamber should be dark and quiet. If outside noise is a problem, try

a white noise machine or one that produces relaxing nature sounds.

- Reserve your bedchamber for sleep. No work, no laptops, no kids. Maybe a book to relax your mind, but that's all.
- If you have a poor night's sleep, don't make it worse by worrying about it. You will have another chance real soon, and worrying will only make it worse.

Commit to sleep as a priority. If you wake up two hours early, don't say, "Well, since I'm up, I may as well get some work done." Lie down, overachiever. Let your body relax, and you'll go back to sleep. You'll get more done in less time if you're fully rested.

The Jack: Managing Stress

The problem here isn't stress in itself, but *continual* stress. We all are visited by stress; life is a stressful state of being. The difference comes in how you manage it. Your body was made to respond to stressful situations in particular ways, and when the stress is sudden and brief, this response is useful. Your sympathetic nervous system goes on alert, and your adrenal glands flood your body with adrenaline and cortisol. This reaction increases blood flow to your brain and muscle and releases stored glucose, so your mind feels more keen, you don't notice pain, and you experience a flood of speed and energy.

The problem comes when you experience the stress response more or less constantly. Modern life regularly conjures up stressful situations: traffic jams, financial trouble, overwork, IRS audits—you name it. Add chronic lack of sleep, throw in a haphazard, on-the-go diet, and you have a recipe for stressed-out skin, hair, and health. When your stress response never truly subsides, your body is constantly reacting to those powerful hormones. This can bring on conditions such as hypertension and skin diseases such as eczema, acne, and rosacea.

The medical world is just beginning to comprehend the health-damaging power of chronic stress. One of its worst effects is on the immune system, which is a structural component of wellness. Chronic stress lowers your T-cell count and makes it harder for your body to fight off infections. From your heart to your brain, unrelieved stress is a vicious enemy of wellness. It's slowly boiling your body from the inside out.

Part of your beauty strategy should be having constructive ways to cope with stress. One of the best is by finding beauty wherever you go. Try teaching yourself to see more beauty around you. Not only can this exercise change your perception of beauty, but also it reduces the body's stress response. Listen to children playing or birds singing, little pleasures that get short shrift when you're racing around. Simply looking at a garden, listening to ocean waves, or stroking a pet can reduce blood pressure. If you can start finding simple beauty in the everyday, you'll never be without a productive way to manage stress.

The other healthy choices we've been talking about are also tip-top for relieving the effects of stress. Get enough sleep, and eat well. Try taking up yoga or meditation. Meditation in particular is a wonder; stacks of research show that it improves chronic pain, arthritis, asthma, premenstrual syndrome, and depression, for starters. It also appears to make regular practitioners more optimistic, and some proponents believe it slows the aging process to help us look fabulous longer.

Over and above those techniques, be good to yourself. Give yourself a break. You're doing great.

BEAUTY BUSTERS

Beauty myths debunked while you wait

Myth: There is such a thing as a healthy suntan.

Fact: *The ladies in the Dutch portraits, with their pale alabaster skin, were on to something: tan-free skin is beautiful. Contrary to popular belief, a suntan does not protect your skin from further sun damage; a suntan is evidence of damage. Over the years, the sun irreversibly damages the elastin fibers in the skin, causing the sagging, wrinkling, and "leather luggage" look that's all too prevalent among seniors who have spent decades in the sun. The major threat, however, is skin cancer. Exposure to ultraviolet (UV) rays causes skin cancer, which is on the rise, with more than one million sun-related nonmelanoma cases diagnosed in the United States each year. For women, melanoma is the most common type of cancer seen between ages twenty-five and thirty, and it's largely caused by sun exposure. There are more than 64,000 new cases in the United States each year—and about 8,000 deaths.*

SPF (which stands for "sun protection factor") ratings identify the level of protection a sunscreen gives you from UVB rays, but now a new "star system" rating system approved by the U.S. Food and Drug Administration makes it easier to choose sunscreens that also provide more protection from UVA rays, which can cause deeper cellular damage. One star means minimal UVA protection, all the way up to four stars for the highest UVA protection available in an over-the-counter product. Still, don't assume that because you have sunscreen on, you can stay out as long as you like. Sunscreen washes off, and UV rays can also cause eye damage. Use SPF clothing or umbrellas to protect yourself. Better yet, play indoors or get your sun exposure early in the morning or in the evening, when the rays are less intense. Also, you're not off the hook if you have dark skin. Even dark skin types need to use sunscreen because of the potential to develop melanoma.

One more thing: early diagnosis is the key to curing melanoma. If you notice a changing mole, a new mole, a dark mole, or a skin lesion that is bleeding or not healing, see your dermatologist immediately. Don't say, "I'll go in a week or two when it's convenient." Go now!

Perfect Ten: Health Care

This last card makes for a winning hand. While women tend to be better on this front than men, we sometimes neglect our health thinking we have to take care of everyone else. NBC's Dr. Nancy Snyderman counsels, "Get yourself off the back burner." See your doctor regularly, get the screenings you should have, and do your self-checks. Since many diseases can be prevented by healthy lifestyle choices, regular visits to your primary care physician can increase your odds of living a long, healthy life. The table on pages 120 and 121 shows the recommended screenings every woman should get.

Among women over age sixty, the rate HIV infection is rising. It may be because older women think that STDs are a young person's disease and that if they're beginning a new relationship after a death or divorce, they don't have to worry about it. We don't know the reasons, but we know the trend. No matter how old you are, practice safe sex.

Seeing your doctor regularly and using good sense changes health care from something stressful to an ongoing relationship, with your health as the goal. Since many diseases, including many

Recommended Health Screenings and Vaccinations

Procedure	Ages 18–39	Ages 40–49	Ages 50–64	Ages 65+
General physical	Annually	Annually	Annually	Twice a year
Thyroid test	Every 5 years starting at age 35	Every 5 years	Every 5 years	Every 5 years
Blood pressure test	At least every 2 years	At least every 2 years	At least every 2 years	At least every 2 years
Cholesterol test	Annually starting at age 20	Annually	Annually	Annually
Bone mineral density test		Discuss with your doctor based on family history	Discuss with your doctor based on family history	Have at least 1 test; repeat based on results
Blood sugar test (for diabetes)	Depends on weight and family history	Every 3 years starting at age 45	Every 3 years	Every 3 years
Mammogram	Depends on family history of breast cancer	Every 1–2 years	Every 1–2 years	Every 1–2 years
Pap test and pelvic exam	Annually if you are sexually active or older than 21	Every 1–3 years	Every 1–3 years	If 3 normal tests and no abnormal tests in 10 years, ask your doctor about stopping

Fecal occult blood test		Every year with annual physical	Every year with annual physical	Every year with annual physical
Colonoscopy			Every 5 years	Every 5 years
Eye exam	If you have vision problems, at least 1 exam from age 20 to 29 and 2 from age 30 to 39	Every 2–4 years	Every 2–4 years	Every 1–2 years
Hearing test	Every 10 years starting at age 18	Every 10 years	Every 10 years	Every 10 years
Skin exam	Monthly mole self-check; physician exam every 3 years starting at age 20	Monthly mole self-check; physician exam every year with annual physical	Monthly mole self-check; physician exam every year with annual physical	Monthly mole self-check; physician exam every year with annual physical
Dental exam	1–2 times a year	1–2 times a year	1–2 times a year	1–2 times a year
Influenza vaccine	Discuss with your doctor	Discuss with your doctor	Annually	Annually
Pneumonia vaccine				1 time only
Tetanus-diphtheria booster	Every 10 years	Every 10 years	Every 10 years	Every 10 years
HPV vaccine	Once, between ages 9 and 26			

cancers, are very treatable when caught early, regular health-care visits are a wonderful way of ensuring that you remain beautiful on the inside—and therefore, on the outside.

The Loop Gets a Workout

We're not going to bore you with the reasons why exercise, sensible diet, and the other basics of good health are beneficial. You've read about them: a strong cardiovascular system, weight control, avoiding osteoporosis and diabetes, and so on. What we will tell you is that other than inner beauty, nothing activates the Beauty-Brain Loop more forcefully than improving your health.

In fact, health is a close cousin of inner beauty. Improving either one sets the loop in motion. For example, when you begin an exercise program, you do more than bolster your self-esteem by looking slimmer. You also spark the infamous "runner's high" by opening the valve to a cascade of serotonin, dopamine, and endorphins, making you feel terrific after a workout. The more you exercise, the better you feel. Just embarking on a concerted, professionally designed program of fitness and nutrition makes you feel more in control and more able to tame your body's stress response and, as you shape up and take on a more attractive profile, gives your self-esteem a sturdy lift.

Eating well also makes you feel well. "Self-esteem absolutely can be affected by being well nourished," dietitian McCune told us in her interview. "A well-nourished brain can make you feel better about yourself, while a poorly nourished brain can result in problems such as hypoglycemia. If you think you can't manage yourself and your life, you're going to feel bad about yourself."

Beyond that, health is a real boon to outer beauty. Both lots of exercise and healthful foods are godsends for your skin, especially when you're consuming plenty of omega-3 and omega-6 fatty acids and antioxidants. And it goes without saying that when you're fit, toned, and at your ideal weight, your clothes fit better, and you look and feel more attractive.

As for environment . . . well, when you're working out and eating like an Olympic athlete, you glow with energy and self-confidence. That's obvious and infectious. If you want to become the center of attention, be at optimum health. When you're serene and self-assured, you are always beautiful. People will respond. Count on it.

MAYBE YOU HADN'T THOUGHT OF . . .

Legendary yoga master B. K. S. Iyengar said, "Health is a state of complete harmony of the body, mind, and spirit. When one is free from physical disabilities and mental distractions, the gates of the soul open." Nothing we've said in this chapter reflects our view more clearly. Health is more than having a strong heart and firm muscles. It's feeling fantastic from your bones to your brain. It's taking stairs three at a time and not caring who notices.

Here are a few more windfalls of healthy habits that you may not have thought about:

- **A fitter brain.** It's easy to overlook how a healthy lifestyle affects this most important of organs. Enjoy knowing that what's good for the rest of your body is also dynamite for your gray matter. Studies show that regular exercise helps the memory center form new neural connections, as well as delivering more oxygen-rich blood to the entire brain. The brain is just like the rest of the body: the more we use it, the better it gets. A heart-healthy diet also keeps the blood vessels that feed your brain clear and elastic, and anything that helps you manage stress, from getting enough sleep to weekly yoga classes or meditation, is also a big plus.

• **Better posture.** When you're out of shape, you slouch. You curve inward on yourself. When you know you're fit, you pull your shoulders and head back. Your chin comes up. Your arms swing firmly. You look and feel better. Correct posture not only looks terrific but also helps prevent falls and the pain caused by using the wrong muscles. Walking properly activates the muscles in your abdomen, thighs, and glutes, so proper posture can actually give you a better rear end, and who doesn't want that?

• **More sex appeal.** Researchers at the University of Arkansas found that men and women reported feeling sexier the more fit they were. Feeling good about your body has benefits in bed and out. Being in shape also gives you more endurance, which is handy during sex.

• **Freedom.** This might be the greatest gift of all. Health frees you—from stereotypes of aging, from limitations on your mobility, from dependency, and from many of the risks of disease and decay.

Free, healthy, and beautiful. That's quite a jackpot. It's within your reach if you play your cards right.

Beauty Bullets

ॐ Health is the foundation of beauty.

ॐ Our DNA attracts us to health because it tells us someone can help us pass on our genes.

ॐ You don't have to be thin to be healthy.

ᛣ There are five cards in your health hand: exercise, nutrition, sleep, stress management, and health care.

ᛣ Being healthy improves all other stages of the Beauty-Brain Loop.

BEAUTY AND THE BRAIN Rx

You Are Getting Sleepy . . .

Dr. Debra: *There are a lot of old wives' tales regarding sleep and the skin, one of which is the idea of the "beauty rest," in which skin repair happens while you're asleep. In reality, the sloughing of skin cells and skin renewal is going on all the time, regardless of when or how much you sleep. However, sleep is critical to general health, and getting seven to eight hours per night (for most women) is a must. Sleep is one of the ways that the body recovers from the effects of stress hormones, so lack of sleep can allow those hormones to slow collagen production in the skin, leading to sagging. Also, sleeplessness can alter blood vessel tone and cause puffiness or bags in the thin skin under the eyes. And because sufficient sleep helps you be healthier overall, it can help you bring out your skin's optimal natural beauty.*

Dr. Eva: *Sleep and mental and emotional health are closely linked. Lack of sleep is a major contributor to irritability, outbursts of anger, and impatience, which can damage your relationships. More seriously, altered sleep patterns can signal depression, anxiety disorders, or bipolar disorder, while chronic sleeplessness is a contributing factor to the development of clinical depression. So, it's important to make sleep a priority for everyone in your family.*

6

Outer Beauty: It's OK to Want to Look Fantastic

*Even beauties can be unattractive. If you catch a
beauty in the wrong light at the right time, forget it.
I believe in low lights and trick mirrors. I believe in
plastic surgery.*

—Andy Warhol

WAITER, COULD WE get the reality check, please? We're physicians. We work hard. We see patients, write articles, teach, and speak. We write books. We have families and teenage kids. We do our best to look our best, but sometimes we're just hanging on for dear life, running to the store in workout clothes and hoping we won't see anyone we know. Odds are you're nodding in recognition, because you do the same thing. We're not living in the fictional world of Stepford, Connecticut. We're just trying to do whatever we can to look beautiful while juggling life's other demands. Sometimes, we succeed. Other times, we just thank our lucky stars that we're not followed by paparazzi. In short, we're like every other professional woman.

Still, perfection beckons. Wanting to look great is more than pride. Looking like the social ideal of beauty may give women a competitive advantage. The closer we are to what our particular culture sees as the ideal female image, the more beautiful others will find us. Beauty isn't just "easy on the eyes"; it also appeases the brain. We like averageness (apologies to Picasso, but no one wants to see a nose on the side of the forehead) and symmetry (both sides of the body balanced). These qualities are just appealing.

Lustrous hair, glowing skin, pearl-white teeth, and a curvaceous figure are advantages in that most primal of competitions, the battle for the perfect mate. As David M. Buss writes in *The Evolution of Desire*, "Women do not compete to communicate accurate information to men. Rather, they compete to activate men's evolved psychological standards of beauty, keyed to youth and health." Because of this innate, hardwired sense of beauty, looking great imparts a competitive edge in every area of life, from jobs to the legal system and beyond. That's why caring about beauty is not the same thing as being vain.

Buss goes on to state that because women evolved with men who desired youth and health in potential mates, we have evolved the motivation to appear young and healthful. So when you have an "Aha!" moment after getting your hair done, it's your genes saying. "You go, girl!"

It's more than OK to want to look beautiful, and this chapter will tell you ways to make the most of what you've got that are smart, healthy, and inexpensive.

THE CANARY IN THE COAL MINE

Until the mid-1900s, mine workers would carry canaries down into the tunnels to detect the presence of deadly methane gas.

If a canary died, it was a warning that the men should evacuate immediately. Your outer beauty is your canary. For better or worse, it's almost impossible to hide the state of your inner beauty or health. Unless you go to ridiculous lengths to conceal the evidence, your outer beauty tells all.

If you're getting enough sleep, eating a healthy diet, and exercising sufficiently, it's going to show in your hair and skin. If you're smoking, failing to protect yourself from the sun, or eating greasy junk, the yellowed teeth or the blemishes of acne will spill your secret to the world. We know a woman close to forty who's a real athlete and is in tremendous physical condition. At first, no one knew that she was suffering from untreated clinical depression; her toned body fooled everyone into thinking she was fine inside and out. Then a neighbor asked her about the heavy dark circles under her eyes. Turns out she hadn't slept well in months and had been self-medicating with alcohol. Fortunately, she got help, but without that outer-beauty canary singing away, no one might have suspected anything until it was too late.

You can't hide from your outer beauty. The skin is a hypersensitive link to your mind, your body, and the outside world. It's also a walking billboard for your health. Traumas, stress, and toxins often announce themselves on the skin before you're aware of them anywhere else. Diseases can manifest first in the mouth as bad breath. Similarly, nutritional deficiencies can take the form of brittle hair or crumbling nails. A new, multidisciplinary field of medical study is suggesting that the skin is almost an intelligent, independent system all its own. And my, does that system talk, revealing everything that's going wrong with your body and mind. If you're neglecting your inner beauty and your health, outer beauty becomes your neighborhood gossip.

OUTER BEAUTY AND THE LOOP

Outer beauty comprises your skin, teeth, hair, nails, fashion style, jewelry, accessories, and anything else that creates the immediate visible package that people see on the street. All the stages of the Beauty-Brain Loop impact these areas, but health tends to speak before the others can get a word in edgewise. Whether you're taking maximal care of your body or living in the fast-food drive-through lane, your appearance will show it quickly and clearly. The older you get, the less forgiving your

---

BEAUTY BUDDIES

Pamela Williams, fifty, and Joy Wheeler, fifty-two

Best friends in Kansas City, Missouri, for more than twenty years, Pam and Joy form a sort of "pampering posse," accompanying each other on high-end shopping sojourns around the city and to destinations such as Cancun, where they take great pleasure in lounging in swimwear.

"We do like to travel together," says Pam, a hospital human resources director. "We're on a vacation together at least once a year. It's not always just the two of us, though it might as well be. It's really our time to get reconnected. That tradition started on the balcony of a time-share in Cancun."

Their most recent trip was to Paris, during which they joined a group of other women to celebrate Pam's fiftieth birthday in style and even adopted French names for the duration. "I chose Amelie, and she was Fifi," Joy says. "I thought this would be a great opportunity to have some girlfriend time with my best friend in Paris, and the tour guide said we should come up with French names because we simply couldn't be walking across Pont Neuf calling each other Pam and Joy."

"It's not about the destination for us; it's the journey that's so much fun," says Pam. "We had a store closed to the public in Venice so they could help us buy jewelry. In Paris, these store owners were serving us champagne while they were altering a skirt for me. It's about the clothing and the jewelry, but what we really love is getting to know the people. It's an adventure."

"We can spend an entire day from morning until night," Joy says. "We go to eat at the latest time possible so we can maximize every hour in the day for our adventure. There's no one else we can do that with. We have that compatibility."

Pam concludes, "It's really about having the confidence to do what you want to do and being comfortable enough in your own skin to do it."

body becomes. Here's how the other parts of the loop affect your outer beauty:

* **Inner beauty.** How you cope with stress determines whether inner beauty is the hero or villain of the piece. Chronic, unrelieved stress devastates the skin, leading to outbreaks and hampering its role as a major part of the immune system, which can lead to more frequent sickness. Also, if you have poor self-esteem, you're more likely to neglect self-care such as sun protection, hairstyling, and dressing well, bringing down your outer beauty.

- **Health.** As we said, health doesn't waste time about announcing itself in your outer beauty. It's pretty logical: if your diet is sensible, and you're fit, you're going to have healthier skin and hair and look better in any clothing.
- **Environment.** The wider world is the ultimate feedback channel for outer beauty. When you look sharp, you hear about it from others; when you don't, you hear a big fat nothing. Either way, the response of your environment (or fear of how it will respond) can motivate you to do what it takes to look your best.

Of course, the current runs both ways. Outer beauty also affects each stage in the loop as well. How attractive you feel and how others react to you can either advance or reverse your

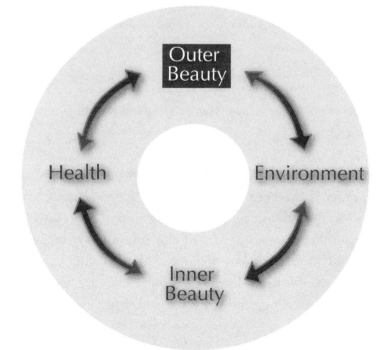

self-esteem; the knowledge that you look hot is a fabulous mood-altering substance. Since our society is so acutely aware of weight, musculature, and overall fitness, the desire to look your best can be powerful fuel to improve your fitness level and live a healthy lifestyle. You don't need a medical degree to know how outer beauty can set your environment on its ear. Just watch a group of men at a gathering when a beautiful woman enters the room: they stop talking all at once.

There's nothing shallow about wanting to be lovely, not when attractiveness wields such influence over the rest of you. However, it is shallow to insist on fitting into some societal standard of beauty. We're always saddened at the prospect of a slender, athletic, pretty but small-breasted young woman getting breast-enlargement surgery because she feels inadequate without the big bosom a hundred magazines tell her she's supposed to have.

We implore every woman to pursue her own brand of beauty, a look that's uniquely hers. Not everyone has a Pam Anderson chest or Elle McPherson legs, but every woman has something about her that's beautiful: bright eyes, a dazzling smile, or maybe the graceful hands of a piano virtuosa. We want to give you the insight and information you need to make the most of what you've got—to be the best you possible. Be *your* kind of beautiful, and leave the desperate beauty stories to the tabloids.

The Distorted Self

The alternative can be not just unhappy but also unhealthy. Some women move beyond obsessing about their looks into mental illness. The woman you know who constantly checks the mirror may not be vain but instead be suffering from body dysmorphic disorder, or BDD. People with this condition (which is thought to affect 1 to 2 percent of the population) fixate on perceived flaws in the face or body. They find themselves checking their appearance in the mirror from three to eight hours every day and continually thinking about their so-called flaws.

Even a beautiful woman with BDD may describe her skin, stomach, or nose as "monstrous." Women suffering from this disorder look in the mirror, see only how they fall short of some beauty ideal, and obsess over the details they believe are responsible. Some may go on to have unnecessary cosmetic surgery, but this fails to address the real issue and sometimes makes the situation even worse while exposing the woman to the expense and risks of surgery. Patients sometimes shop around from doctor to doctor trying to find a solution to the perceived problem. Psychotherapy and sometimes medication will help women suffering from BDD, but changing their appearance doesn't help. Such women often curtail their social lives and develop depression or anxiety disorders.

How you interpret the events and people in your life has a lot to do with your risk for developing BDD, as well as depression or anxiety. Researchers have found that patients with BDD have a decreased ability to identify their own emotional expressions and so were also more likely to misinterpret other people's emotions. They were more apt to believe that others were rejecting them, reinforcing their distorted view of themselves. Healthy ways of interpreting and explaining life's vicissitudes are integral to strong inner beauty.

The Artist's Tools

If a beautiful woman is a work of art (and we certainly agree that's the case), then the aspects that create outer beauty are each pieces in the artist's toolkit. Let's sort through the various tools a woman can use to create the masterpiece that is herself.

For each, the vital principles are maintenance and protection. Every part of your outer beauty, from skin to teeth, thrives when you're proactive—taking steps to ensure vitality before there's a problem—and when you get preventive, whether it's wearing sunscreen or getting your teeth cleaned every six months. Long-term thinking can go a long way to preventing short-term quick fixes—and the big price tags that come with them.

Skin: Your Canvas

This book really did begin as a conversation between us as we lounged under an umbrella on a Jamaican beach, taking a well-deserved break from our practices. With our skin covered in protective sunscreen and looking out over the turquoise surf, we chatted about how the sun aged skin and then about aging and the anxiety women feel concerning it. This eventually led us to compare patients and note how many factors they had in common: self-esteem issues related to appearance, pressure from a beauty-obsessed culture, and the need for guidance to make smart and healthy choices about their inner and outer beauty. Thus, a book was born from a talk about skin.

We hope we have convinced you that looking youthful and healthy for as long as possible is the best beauty not-so-secret secret. When you look at people, how do you judge their age? Most of the information comes from looking at the skin. So, when it comes to beauty, your skin is the asset that should get your utmost attention and protection.

Your skin is three layers of amazing biological engineering that's gauze-thin but tough as nails, absorbing moisture, protecting you from the elements, and regulating your body temperature. It's the first line of defense of your immune system and the source of tactile contact with the world. Skin comes in five basic types:

- **Normal:** You don't have a tendency to break out and don't need moisturizer daily. Lucky you.
- **Oily:** Your skin appears shiny, and you break out frequently because your sebaceous glands produce excessive oil. You need to use degreasing cleansers and sometimes masks to absorb the excess.
- **Dry:** No matter how much moisturizer you put on, you're always dry and cracking, and your skin feels tight. Washing with nonsoap, moisturizing cleansers is the way to go.
- **Sensitive:** Anything you put on your skin causes you to break out or get a rash. This necessitates products designed for sensitive skin.
- **Combination:** Up to half of women have this type of skin, with oily skin typically on the forehead and nose, and normal or dry skin elsewhere. Your cleansing routine needs to be customized for your different areas.

Skin is easy to take for granted, isn't it? Maybe that's because our skin is a common denominator through every life stage: silky baby and toddler skin, acne-ridden adolescent skin, decorated skin in our mate-finding twenties and thirties, pampered skin as we edge cautiously into our forties and beyond, and sagging and sun-damaged skin in the sixties and beyond. It's one of the parts of the body that betray our age. No matter how hard we work at the health club to stay fit and trim into our seventies or eighties, our skin will still become thinner, drier, and old-looking. Maybe we neglect our skin to get back at it: "I'll show you, making me look like an old lady! How about a dose of solar radiation, Scarecrow?"

Remember that your skin is truly the canvas on which all other aspects of your outer beauty are painted. As any artist knows, without a good canvas on which to work, even the most

---

✑ BEAUTY STORY: "JUDY"

Judy, forty-one, came to Debra's office suffering from hirsutism, an excess of body and facial hair. This condition can be caused by hormonal abnormalities but is also more common in people with a certain genetic background, typically Middle Eastern or Mediterranean descent. Judy was depressed and embarrassed by her condition, which manifested on her face, arms, and chest. She was forced to shave every day, which made her feel unfeminine. She favored masculine clothing because she was afraid to show her chest and would not wear tank tops or bathing suits because of the hair on her arms. Debra recommended laser hair removal to treat large areas. After monthly treatment for eight months, Judy now has 80 percent permanent hair reduction, meaning she does not have excessive growth in those areas. She now wears more feminine clothing, and her self-esteem is markedly improved.

Eva: *Body image dictates how we view ourselves. We look in the mirror and can allow our image to tell us how feminine or masculine we are. Our inner critic can be so harsh that our self-esteem suffers. It seems that was the case with Judy. Freeing her from the hair allowed her self-esteem to soar.*

Debra: *She was beautiful, but she couldn't see it. All she could see was the hair. We're raised to believe that women's skin should be smooth and flawless. That's why the development of more facial hair after menopause can be jarring for some women, and genetic hirsutism can seem like a curse.*

deft brushstrokes are wasted. When you're seeking to maximize your outer beauty, start by taking care of your skin the way it takes care of you.

A COLLAGEN EDUCATION. For women, our skin puts us at a disadvantage from the start. We have thinner skin than men, which makes us more likely to dry out and suffer sun damage. In menopause, the loss of both estrogen and testosterone increases the breakdown of collagen, slows the sloughing and replacement of dead cells, and accentuates crow's-feet and the "marionette" lines between the nose and chin. Even if you're genetically blessed, keeping your skin healthy and beautiful into later life is hard work.

Your skin is a wonder consisting of three layers:

1. **Epidermis:** This outer layer is made up of several layers of cells, the majority being keratinoctyes. These cells migrate upward through the epidermis, and by the time they reach the surface of your skin, they have become more rigid and form a protective barrier.

2. **Dermis:** This is the skin's business district. The serious infrastructure of your skin is woven through the dermis: hair follicles, blood vessels, nerve fibers, sebaceous glands that produce your skin's oil, sweat glands, and the collagen and elastin that support your skin. As you can imagine, a lot happens in the dermis. This layer delivers water and nutrients to the epidermis, keeping it healthy. This is where stress sets off excess production of oil in the sebaceous glands, sparking acne outbreaks. It's where intense emotion causes a rush of blood to the skin, producing a blush. The sweat that drips off you during an aerobics class? Manufactured here.

The foundation of the dermis—and one of the foundations of beautiful skin—is collagen. This protein, which makes up about one-third of all the protein in the body, forms about 95 percent of the dermis. Together with elastin, it creates the basic structure for your skin, an organic woven framework on which skin cells thrive. The healthier your collagen, the firmer and springier your skin. As we age, collagen begins to break down faster than the body can replace it. Skin sags, and wrinkles appear. One solution is a new generation of injectable fillers that show promising results. More on these in Chapter 10.

3. Subcutaneous layer: This is a layer of mostly fat of varying thicknesses that contains larger blood vessels and contributes to skin firmness. As with collagen, it's lost somewhat as we age. Babies' cheeks are so pinchingly plump because they're loaded with healthy collagen and fat.

THE USUAL SUSPECTS. There's that word again: *age*. Age affects every part of our bodies, but its effects become most visible to others through that very visible canvas. While we can sure-enough age the rest of our bodies prematurely through poor lifestyle choices, nowhere is this more apt to occur than with our skin. There are two types of skin aging: *extrinsic*, which comes from external factors, and *intrinsic*, which is genetic.

If there's a mustache-twisting bad guy in the police lineup of extrinsic factors, it's the sun. Forget the "But what about vitamin D?" excuse. You can get all the vitamin D you need from fifteen minutes in the sun. Beyond that, if you're unprotected, you're just doing damage. Sun damage, or photoaging, is the main cause of premature skin aging and the target of more than 90 percent of skin therapies. That's billions of dollars spent each year in the United States to repair damage that's totally preventable through smart choices.

The most common forms of sun damage are related to melanin, the skin pigmentation produced by melanocytes. Melanin protects the skin to some extent from sun damage, but overexposure to the sun produces brown or red discolorations, commonly called "age spots" (they really should be called "sunspots," but the astronomers took that one). Hyperpigmentation is one of the most frequent complaints of women seeking therapy from a dermatologist or an aesthetician. (Note: A dermatologist is a physician who specializes in the skin; an aesthetician is a licensed cosmetology professional who is not a doctor.)

Of more immediate concern is the damage ultraviolet rays do to the skin. UV rays, both the A and B wavelengths, break down the supporting collagen and elastin, causing wrinkles, sagging, the classic "leathery" skin that comes from years of suntanning, and, of course, skin cancers. Contrary to what you might have heard, tanning beds are not a safe alternative; they produce heavy doses of UVA radiation that age the skin and can increase the risk of cancers. Not to mention that women report getting diseases such as herpes from unhygienic tanning beds, reason enough to steer clear of the places, in our opinion.

Sun isn't the only culprit in our lineup, though. All right, step forward when we call your name . . .

- **Smoking:** Tobacco smoke reduces the oxygen supply to the skin, resulting in lower collagen and elastin production. It also breaks down an enzyme that controls collagen production.
- **Stress:** Relentless stress makes your whole body feel rotten, and your skin can show it. Stress is a common cause of acne outbreaks, while sleep deprivation, which frequently goes hand-in-

hand with stressful situations, contributes to eye bags and eyelid sagging.

- **Poor diet:** Start a crash diet to drop weight fast, and it will show in your sagging skin. More generally, a poor diet or yo-yo dieting can deprive your skin of the antioxidants, vitamins, and minerals it needs to stay healthy.
- **Alcohol:** Excessive drinking leads to enlargement of the blood vessels, dehydration, and a sallow complexion, sometimes producing spider veins and the classic drinker's broken veins around the nose.

Intrinsic aging stems from that pesky DNA again. You don't have much control over this (yet), but looking at your parents can give you some hint of what's in store for your skin. If your

BEAUTY PEARLS

I think that a woman's true beauty is on the inside. As president and visionary of the Cancer Schmancer Movement, I encourage all women to know what ingredients are in their skin-care products. The skin is the biggest organ in the body, yet there is no FDA standard for the products we use to look beautiful. Currently, the cosmetics industry is self-regulated, essentially the fox guarding the henhouse. Log on to the Compact Alliance as well as Safe Cosmetics and see what these groups consider carcinogen-free products. Let's all try to make an effort to apply safer skin-care products so that what makes us beautiful on the outside also keeps us beautiful on the inside.

—Fran Drescher, president and visionary of the
Cancer Schmancer Movement
Author, actor, uterine cancer survivor

mother's skin aged excessively from moderate sun exposure, for instance, there's a good chance you inherited a genetic factor that makes your skin more vulnerable to photoaging. In that case, you may be able to prevent extra damage by making smart lifestyle choices now.

THE VAMPIRE STRATEGY. The face is the front line of the aging-skin war as we do close combat with droopy eyelids, age spots, lines, and wrinkles. Signs of aging also make themselves known in other areas, most notably the neck, chest, and hands. The neck can sag with age, creating bands of wrinkled skin or neck wattles. Skin on the chest is extremely thin and often exposed, and it's not uncommon to see older women who've spent a lot of time in the sun with crepey, blotchy, wrinkled skin in their décolletage. The hands are exposed not only to the sun but also to chemicals such as those in dish-washing soap and bleach, often resulting in wrinkles and visible blood vessels.

So, what's to be done? First of all, adopt what we call the "vampire strategy": stay out of the sun. Protect your skin from the sun's rays when you're outdoors. This requires just a little attention and planning, but it's hard to get some women, especially young women, to take sun protection seriously. It's never too early to start wearing a "broad-spectrum" SPF 15–30 sunscreen, one that protects against UVA and UVB rays; avoiding sun exposure between ten A.M. and two P.M. during the summer; and wearing protective clothing and hats. Be sure to reapply your sunscreen every two to three hours. If you live in a region where the sun is more intense, bump the SPF to 30–45.

The easiest way to ensure that you're always protected is to apply a daily moisturizer with a built-in sunscreen. To help remember your sunscreen daily, keep it at your sink. In the morning after brushing your teeth, immediately apply your sunscreen. And if you simply must have a tan, get one that comes from a bottle.

Other basic ways to prevent excessive aging of the skin are also no-brainers: cleanse your skin every morning with a product that's appropriate to your skin type, drink six to eight glasses of water daily, and eat a diet that's rich in omega-3 fatty acids (salmon, mackerel, albacore tuna, or 1,000-milligram daily supplements) and antioxidants (brightly colored fruits and vegetables, berries, green tea, and nuts rich in selenium and zinc). Get lots of sleep, exercise regularly, and try calming disciplines such as yoga, tai chi, or nature hikes.

Other skin antiaging options range from simple supplements and home products to in-office procedures that should be done only by a physician:

- **Supplements:** Consider taking folic acid, magnesium, and calcium, as well as omega-3s, coenzyme Q10, and alpha lipoic acid, a powerful anti-inflammatory agent. Always consult your doctor before starting a supplement regimen.
- **Moisturizers:** If you have oily skin, you may not need moisturizer. For others, used regularly, effective moisturizers protect the skin while sealing in moisture.
- **Cosmeceuticals:** Some new lotions and creams contain therapeutic ingredients such as peptides, growth factors, or antioxidants.
- **Antioxidants:** Antioxidants such as vitamins A, C, and E and beta-carotene help prevent cellular damage from external forces, such as pollution, cigarette smoke, and the sun, and from inter-

nal forces, such as stress hormones and the normal oxidation of food. They are a trusty antiaging ally.

• **Peptides:** These chains of amino acids (the building blocks of proteins) help stimulate the skin's natural rebuilding process by facilitating communication between the skin's layers.

• **Retinoids:** Retin-A and Renova are commonly used prescription topicals containing vitamin A derivatives that stimulate collagen production, balance skin tone, and reduce dark spots from photoaging. For people who are sensitive, there are some well-tolerated over-the-counter retinol products. Women who are pregnant or nursing should avoid retinoids.

• **Bleaching creams:** These can reduce age spots, treat melasma (dark facial skin coloration), and brighten the skin. Prescription preparations tend to be more effective than OTC products and often contain ingredients such as hydroquinone, an organic skin bleaching compound (examples: Triluma, Lustra, Epiquin).

• **Botox:** The most popular cosmetic procedure in the United States (done more than three million times a year), Botox uses botulinum toxin to reduce facial muscle contractions that produce forehead lines and wrinkles.

• **Dermal fillers:** Ranging from collagen to hyaluronic acid (the skin's natural moisturizing agent), fillers are injected under the skin to reduce the appearance of nasolabial folds (the lines that run from the nose to the corners of the mouth) and wrinkles.

• **Physical exfoliation:** Microdermabrasion is a manual exfoliation technique that removes the dead cells that often clog the outer layers of the skin, stimulating collagen production and new cell growth.

• **Chemical peels or chemical exfoliation:** Commonly done using alpha hydroxy acids and beta hydroxy acids (natural acids in dairy products, sugar, and citrus fruits), chemical peels unclog

---

BEAUTY BUSTERS

Beauty myths debunked while you wait

Myth: Dryness causes wrinkles.

Fact: Dryness and dehydration have nothing to do with causing wrinkles. Wrinkles result from the breakdown of the collagen and elastin fibers that form the structural support for skin cells. The causes of this damage are not dryness but age, nutritional deficiencies, and, most commonly, overexposure to the sun. Overexposure to solar radiation denatures the protein that makes up collagen. It's like putting your skin in a microwave oven.

The upshot is that, contrary to what commercials may tell you, moisturizers do nothing to prevent or repair wrinkles. They can temporarily trap moisture in the skin, but that's all. If you want to prevent wrinkles, you should avoid sun exposure and eat a diet rich in antioxidants, phytonutrients, and omega-3 fatty acids. You may also want to use a moisturizing lotion that contains alpha hydroxy acids (which encourage collagen growth) and exfoliate dead skin cells once or twice a week, stimulating new cell growth. Also add skin-care products with retinol, which can stimulate new collagen.

Repairing wrinkles means using injectable fillers or Botox, procedures that last for up to nine months.

---

pores and remove damaged epidermal layers, making them effective for treating mild hyperpigmentation, acne, and wrinkles. For more serious skin problems, peels can also be done using trichloroacetic acid, which is stronger.

• **Intense pulse light:** Also known as photorejuvenation, this procedure uses light to treat brown spots, broken capillaries, and rosacea and to tighten pores.

• **Photodynamic therapy:** This remedy for extreme sun damage and precancers uses Levulin, a topical solution applied to the skin, prior to treatment with a laser or intense pulse light.

• **Lasers:** A multitude of lasers can treat various skin problems. For antiaging, there are nonablative lasers (Cooltouch), minimally ablative lasers (erbium, or Laser Peel), and ablative lasers (CO_2). Ablation refers to removing the top layers of the skin.

• **Fractional skin resurfacing:** This procedure, which uses a laser to produce thousands of tiny, deep columns in the skin, is a treatment for acne scars, brown spots, fine wrinkles, and melasma. Fraxel and Affirm are examples.

• **Radio-frequency treatments:** Avoid the knife with devices such as Thermage, which uses radio waves to revitalize collagen and elastin, tightening the skin.

• **Infrared-based tightening procedures:** Titan is an example of this technology that uses infrared radiation to heat collagen, causing the skin to contract.

DR. DEBRA'S DAILY BEAUTIFUL SKIN REGIMEN. In Chapter 8, we talk about the kinds of cosmetic procedures you may want to consider through the decades to come, but great skin begins with daily care, and that's what we're going to give you here. The rule is simple: the better care you take of your skin today, the fewer expensive procedures you're likely to need tomorrow. By keeping it simple, you'll have a skin regimen that works and that you can stick to.

The Appendix, "Shopping the Beauty Counter with Dr. Debra," walks you through the best brands in each of the major skin-care product categories, together with what they cost.

If you're age twenty to thirty . . .

Daily A.M. regimen	Step 1	Step 2
Oily skin	Wash with a glycolic or salicylic acid cleanser	Apply an SPF 15–30 broad-spectrum oil-free sunscreen
Dry skin	Wash with a gentle, nonsoap cleanser	Apply an SPF 15–30 broad-spectrum sunscreen with moisturizer
Regular/ combination skin	Wash with a mild glycolic or exfoliating cleanser	Apply an SPF 15–30 broad-spectrum sunscreen with moisturizer

Daily P.M. regimen	Step 1	Step 2	Step 3
Oily skin	Wash with a glycolic or salicylic acid cleanser	Use an oil-free, salicylic-based lotion, retinol, or benzoyl peroxide lotion	If breakouts are not controlled, consider prescription nighttime topicals or oral medications
Dry skin	Wash with a nonsoap cleanser	Apply a vitamin- and antioxidant-rich moisturizing cream	
Regular/ combination skin	Wash with a mild glycolic or exfoliating cleanser	Apply a vitamin- and antioxidant-rich, water-based night lotion	

Weekly		
Oily skin	Use a mud or sulfur mask or home microdermabrasion treatment	
Dry skin	Use a glycerin- or oil-based moisturizing mask	

(continued)

Weekly *(cont'd)*	
Regular/ combination skin	Use a *mild* home peel or microdermabrasion treatment

Bimonthly	
All skin types	Apply a beta or alpha hydroxy home peel or mushroom-extract peel

If you're age thirty to forty . . .

Daily A.M. regimen	Step 1	Step 2
Oily skin	Wash with a glycolic or salicylic acid cleanser	Apply an SPF 15–30 broad-spectrum oil-free sunscreen
Dry skin	Wash with a gentle, nonsoap cleanser	Apply an SPF 15–30 broad-spectrum sunscreen with moisturizer
Regular/ combination skin	Wash with a mild glycolic or exfoliating cleanser	Apply an SPF 15–30 broad-spectrum sunscreen with moisturizer

Daily P.M. regimen	Step 1	Step 2	Step 3
Oily skin	Wash with a glycolic or salicylic acid cleanser	Apply a retinol gel or lotion, a benzoyl peroxide lotion, or a salicylic acid lotion	Apply a nighttime eye cream
Dry skin	Wash with a gentle, nonsoap cleanser	Apply a vitamin- and antioxidant-rich moisturizing cream	Apply a nighttime eye cream
Regular/ combination skin	Wash with a mild glycolic or exfoliating cleanser	Apply a vitamin- and antioxidant-rich, water-based night lotion	Apply a nighttime eye cream

Bimonthly*		
All skin types	Use a home peel or microdermabrasion treatment	

If you're over forty . . .

Daily A.M. regimen	Step 1	Step 2
Oily skin	Wash with a glycolic or salicylic acid cleanser	Apply an SPF 15–30 broad-spectrum oil-free sunscreen with antioxidants or growth factor; peptide lotion can be added to decrease the appearance of wrinkles
Dry skin	Wash with a gentle, nonsoap cleanser	Apply an SPF 15–30 broad-spectrum sunscreen with moisturizer and antioxidants or growth factor, plus peptide cream
Sensitive skin	Wash with a gentle, nonsoap cleanser	Apply a chemical-free SPF 15–30 broad-spectrum sunscreen
Regular/ combination skin	Wash with a mild glycolic or exfoliating cleanser	Apply an SPF 15–30 broad-spectrum sunscreen with moisturizer and antioxidants or growth factor, plus peptide cream

Daily P.M. regimen	Step 1	Step 2**	Step 3
Oily skin	Wash with a glycolic or salicylic acid cleanser	Apply a retinol gel	Apply a nighttime eye cream
Dry skin	Wash with a gentle, nonsoap cleanser	Apply a cream with antioxidants and peptides	Apply a nighttime eye cream

(continued)

Daily P.M. regimen *(cont'd)*	Step 1	Step 2**	Step 3
Sensitive skin	Wash with a gentle, nonsoap cleanser	Apply an antioxidant lotion	Apply nighttime eye cream
Regular/ combination skin	Wash with a mild glycolic or exfoliating cleanser	Apply an antioxidant cream or lotion and a retinol cream or lotion	Apply a nighttime eye cream
Bimonthly*			
Oily, dry, or combination skin	Use a home peel or microdermabrasion treatment; if you have rosacea, consult with your dermatologist first		

* If you have persistent acne or rosacea, consider seeing a dermatologist, who can prescribe topical or oral medications that may be more effective for your condition. Always consult with a dermatologist about additional prescription medications that may be available for antiaging or acne.

** If you have brown spots, add application of a bleaching cream to Step 2.

*** If you have wrinkles, consult your dermatologist for prescription-strength retinoid cream. If you have sun damage, your dermatologist can prescribe combination and prescription-strength bleaching creams to add to your regimen.

For Want of a Nail

Beyond skin, other aspects of outer beauty also need your attention, and your nails are one of them. Having your nails done is a healthy social experience, as we already discussed. Being around other women is beneficial to body and mind. To supplement salon services, self-care of the nails is necessary, since people are often judged by the appearance of their hands.

Your fingernails and toenails consist of the protein keratin, which grows from the living tissue in your nail bed. Your nails not only protect your fingertips but also are an excellent vehicle

BEAUTY PEARLS

My cuisine features many immunity enhancing elements essential to preserving good health and preventing disease. These same ingredients also offer many benefits for skin, hair, and nails. My mother and grandmother passed along to me many beauty secrets that they received from their mothers and grandmothers. One of my favorites—and my daughters as well—has kept my skin healthy and clear over the years (see recipe that follows). I also eat a lot of mustard greens, daikon, and zucchini; according to Vietnamese culinary traditions, these are essential to maintain a rosy complexion. And eating turmeric after pregnancy brings back a glowing complexion. Just sauté turmeric and scallions in a little bit of olive oil, and it's delicious and very effective. I also eat a lot of dill, which give me beautiful and strong nails.

—Helen An, founder and chef, Crustacean Restaurant

Recipe: *Chop a few slices of cucumber until they have a fluid consistency. Add 1 teaspoon olive and honey and 1 tablespoon of moisturizer (one with no chemicals if possible). Mix well and put in fridge for a half an hour. Before bed massage into skin and leave on 15 minutes, then rinse off and have sweet dreams!*

for such adornments as polish and decorative appliqués. They are an effective gauge of your overall health as well. Brittle nails can result from vitamin deficiencies, peeling nails can indicate thyroid disease, and crumbling nails can be caused by a fungal infection in the nail bed.

If you can afford it, one of the best ways to care for your nails is to get a professional manicure and pedicure every two to four weeks. In any salon setting, be sure that all the tools are sterilized, or take your own along. As for the procedure itself, do not let the manicurist push back cuticles or clip them. Cuticles serve to protect the nail and the underlying skin from infection. Also watch out for the water! Before soaking your hands or feet, make sure the basin is disinfected.

Here are other nail-care tips for between trips to the salon:

- Keep your hands clean. This helps prevent fungal and bacterial infections and nail discoloration. Wash with mild soap.
- If you work out and shower at a gym, wear shower shoes to avoid picking up a fungal infection.
- Trim your nails regularly if you don't wear them long. Trim toenails straight across to avoid ingrown toenails.
- Avoid biting your nails. If you're a habitual nail chewer, try some of the antibiting nail polish out there. It's nasty tasting but effective.

 ## BEAUTY BOOSTERS

Practical things you can do now to be more beautiful

You can enhance your attractiveness to others simply by making eye contact and smiling when you're in a social situation. The same studies showing that beautiful faces activate the brain's reward circuitry also show that making eye contact and smiling enhance the intensity of the reward provided. So, by looking directly into the eyes of people to whom you're speaking (regardless of gender) and smiling as they speak, and even by looking into their eyes as you shake hands upon meeting, you make being near you more rewarding. This simple approach enhances your inner beauty and lets your outer beauty be more fully appreciated.

- Eat a healthy diet with plenty of lean protein. Nails are made of protein, and a diet deficient in it will affect nail health.
- Take 2.5 milligrams of biotin daily, which has been shown to produce firmer, harder nails that are more chip-resistant.
- Wear properly fitting shoes to avoid toenail damage.

For tips and ideas on doing your own polish and nail grooming at home, talk to a professional manicurist.

From Hair to Eternity

After the skin, nothing plays up a woman's beauty like her hair. Hair is usually the first thing people notice, and it sends powerful signals to our innate beauty sense as well. Men tend to like shiny objects, including shiny hair. The adage that gentlemen prefer blondes seems to be true, based on the fact that women for hundreds of years have been trying to lighten their hair. Maybe men—and therefore women—like blonde hair because it accompanies lighter skin, which is easier to read for signs of sexual excitement and of health and fertility status. Perhaps blonde hair is a signal of youthfulness and therefore more fertility. Brunettes needn't get discouraged, though, since they have the monopoly on shine.

Hairstyle is highly personal. The best style for you depends on where you are in life, your personality, and even your profession. There's a reason American consumers spend more than $7 billion a year on hair-care products: your hair is the frame for your face, one that can be transformed in an hour to change your entire look. Considering it's dead tissue just like our fingernails, we pay a lot of attention to our manes.

You have either too much hair or too little, and it's in one of three phases at any time: growing, resting, or falling out. As with skin, some shedding is normal; you need to make room for new, healthy hair strands. When you're under stress, though, instead of losing a normal one hundred hairs a day, you might lose two or three times that many, a condition called telogen effluvium. Fortunately, this will correct itself once the source of the stress is gone.

Baldness may be a male stereotype, but many women lose some of their hair at some point in life owing to stress, hormonal factors, or just plain genetics. You could also lose some hair after pregnancy or after stopping birth control. In addition, women who constantly pull their hair back tightly into a bun or ponytail can experience what's called "traction hair loss."

Hair is protein that sprouts from the rich, healthy (ideally) tissue of the scalp, where the follicles and oil-producing glands reside. Even though hair is dead, it can take on all kinds of forms and suffer all kinds of damage—and since it can't heal, the only way to deal with damaged hair is to cut it off, as you know if you've ever had to live with a last-resort "cut-it-off" repair job until it grew out.

There's a lot you can do to keep both hair strands and the scalp healthy, starting with understanding the different types of hair. There are four basic distinguishing characteristics, each with its own gradings:

- **Texture:** Hair can be coarse, fine, or medium. Coarse hair is harder to style or color than the others.
- **Density:** The density of your hair—thin, medium, or thick—has a lot to do with what styles work for you.
- **Wave:** Straight, curly, or coiled? African Americans frequently have coiled hair.

- **Oil:** Finally, your tresses can be dry, normal, or oily. Dry hair usually needs moisturizing products, while oily hair needs products free of oil-adding conditioners.

TRESS FOR SUCCESS. We all want the kind of luxuriant, silky hair we see on television, but getting there takes care and planning. Hair is always exposed to the elements and environmental threats, including UV light, smoke, wind, saltwater, chlorine, and pollution. On top of that, using the wrong care products can dry out and damage hair. Endless coloring, bleaching, and other harsh treatments can fry the cuticle, the outer layer of the strand, leaving it dull or frizzy.

Everything starts with health. Healthy hair is easier to transform into beautiful hair, and it radiates the kind of overall feeling of wellness that's tonic for your self-esteem. So, what can you do to get and keep hair healthy and looking smashing? Some tips:

- **Know your shampoo and conditioner.** The right product for you depends on your hair type. Dry hair needs shampoo with moisturizer, while fine or oily hair needs lightweight products with protein to add body. Hair damaged by sun exposure or chemicals definitely needs conditioner, again suited to your specific type. Keep in mind that your hair will become less oily with age.
- **Condition every time you wash your hair.** This way, you return moisture stripped by UV, chlorine, and other enemies.
- **Don't blow-dry if you don't have to.** Squeeze the water out of your hair, and let it air-dry if you can. If you must blow-dry, use a low setting and shampoo or conditioner that offers thermal protection.

• **Use hair tools with rounded, smooth teeth.** Rough tools can snag and tear the hair fibers.

• **Wear a hat.** Just as it does on your skin, the sun does a number on your hair. Ultraviolet light can break down the protein, leaving hair weak, damage-prone, and dehydrated. You can also use hair products containing sunscreen.

BEAUTY PEARLS

Women wash their hair far too often. We've become addicted to the next best shampoo or conditioner, thinking it'll be the answer for problem hair. Oftentimes, a little of your own natural oil is all you need. Also, trying to attain the unattainable is a huge problem with men and women. If you have three hairs on your head, you're just not going to look like Brigitte Bardot.

The most important part of what makes a woman beautiful is feeling confident, which can't be done with roots six shades darker than your ends unless you live with your hairdresser. Shine is also a huge part of beautiful hair. Once hair has been overprocessed, it's impossible to keep it shiny. Finally, having the right cut means everything. It is extremely important to pay attention to your face shape while choosing a haircut. If you have a wide, round face, don't cut a bob that ends at your chin!

If I had to give women one piece of advice on hair, it would be embrace your natural texture. Stop trying to change it! So many people rely on a flat iron to make their hair something it isn't, and over time they're just destroying the most important part of beautiful hair: health. The same goes for color. Try to stick within a few shades of your natural color. If you have black hair, chances are your skin tone is a good match for it. Of course, adding subtle, "natural" highlights to any color looks beautiful.

—Ruby Weiser, hairstylist

• **Go easy on perms, coloring, and other chemical treatments.** Too much of this can not only wreck your hair but also actually damage your scalp and hinder the growth of new, healthy hair.

As always, you also have to look after your general health. Hair, as with nails, speaks volumes when you're eating a diet deficient in nutrients, especially healthy protein. Eat in balance, and manage stress, and your hair will show it, however it's styled. Here's our advice about styling: find a skilled stylist whom you trust, and stick with him or her. The right cut, color, and highlights are like an instant new look that can make you feel younger or like a vibrant new version of yourself.

Grin and Bare It

When you speak, people's attention veers from your eyes to your mouth. This puts your teeth center stage, so they'd better be looking good. Many women are sensitive about the color and appearance of teeth stained by smoking, coffee, wine, or other foods—so much so that they don't smile or go out in public much due to embarrassment. Poor dental hygiene can also bring on bad breath, another major social taboo.

It's not necessary for anyone to become a hermit. Today, there's a dazzling array of ways to improve the health and appearance of the pearly whites, not all of them expensive.

This isn't just a matter of a white smile. Dental health is strongly linked to overall health. "People don't realize how the health of the oral cavity affects the overall health of our bodies," says Gina Marcus, D.M.D., a cosmetic dentist in Coral Gables, Florida. "It has implications for diabetes, cardiovascular disease, and beyond. The gums and bone underlying the teeth relate very closely to the health of the body. Yet, when you reach certain points in your life, you know you're supposed to do certain things medically, but we don't have the same idea dentally. That's unfortunate, because gastrointestinal cancers often present first in the mouth. A lot of disease is spotted by dentists first."

The basics of dental care are, well, basic. Floss, brush, and rinse (in that order) at home at least twice a day, definitely before going to bed. See your dentist for an exam and cleaning twice a year. Avoid foods heavy in sugar, don't smoke, and go easy on foods that stain teeth, such as red wine and blueberries. You know the drill (pardon the pun) even if you don't do them all.

That's fine as far as it goes, but what if your dental problems are more serious? What if years of neglect have left your teeth misshapen and discolored? There's hope, says Marcus, and attending to the problem is important. "Your smile has such an effect on your self-esteem. For some women, it's all about the size of your breasts or how you look in jeans, but for others, their smile is everything," she says.

"I had a patient once who had serious tetracycline staining on her teeth," she continues. "Nothing worked. She never smiled. She was morose because she felt ugly. I suggested veneers. We did six veneers and a makeover on her, and I have never seen a woman smile more."

For quick fixes, Marcus recommends regular cleanings, during which you can have stains removed and chipped edges on the teeth filed off. She also recommends in-office whitenings, which are cost-effective and make a difference in the appearance of teeth very quickly. If you're on a budget, home whitening products can help, though they are not as strong as in-office techniques.

Other dental solutions to consider:

- **Orthodontia:** With clear braces such as Invisalign, you can have straight teeth minus the social stigma of old-fashioned braces. Average cost: about $5,000.
- **Bonding:** Fill gaps and imperfections in one appointment. Average cost: $300 to $600 per tooth.
- **Gum contouring and grafting:** This procedure reshapes your gums and repairs damage from overbrushing. Average cost: $650 to $850.
- **Tooth contouring:** Minor reshaping of the teeth helps to remove ridges, breaks, chips, and the like. Average cost: $50 to $350 per tooth, depending on how much reshaping is needed.

"If a woman wants to feel better about herself," says Marcus, "doing something with her teeth is a great quick fix. Talk to your dentist, have your teeth cleaned, and see what options are available."

The Colors on Your Palette

Makeup is the paint on your canvas, and it's up to you to decide whether you're Andy Warhol or Claude Monet. There are a hundred great books out there about making yourself look incredible with proper application of makeup, facials, and more. Since we're doctors, our main concern is health. So, let's spend a minute or two on using makeup (and fragrance) in healthy ways. Before we start, though, don't forget the lip gloss or lipstick. They are the number one cosmetic product out there based on sales, and they will set off your winning smile and let your inner beauty shine through.

First and foremost, find the right makeup for your skin type, especially when you're looking for foundation. You'll come across liquid foundations, stick foundations, cream foundations, cream-to-powder foundations, powder compact foundations . . . the choices go on. Each has unique properties, and each comes with a different price tag, depending on the manufacturer. Heavy, pore-clogging foundations are old hat, so select something that will let your skin breathe while protecting it. Some other basic advice:

• **Consult a makeup artist.** Learn what shades, textures, and tools are best for your particular face shape, skin type, and age. Talk to a pro, and get personalized recommendations. To find out about makeup artists who are not affiliated with one cosmetics company, ask at your local beauty salon. Makeup artists generally charge by the hour, and rates can vary widely depending on where you are located and how busy the artist is. So be sure to ask a lot of questions.

• **Try everything before you buy.** Foundation, for example, should melt into your skin with nary a trace, but you can't know if it will by looking at the bottle. Try all your cosmetics on in natural light before you buy them.

• **Care for your skin daily.** You need healthy skin to look your best in your makeup. Follow a daily regimen that includes cleansing with a nonsoap product, applying sunscreen before you go out, moisturizing if you are dry (lightweight during the day, heavier at night for all-night hydration), and applying nighttime eye cream. Exfoliators and masks are handy occasional additions for when you want to clean your pores or remove dead skin. For exfoliation, look for home peels that are gentle and contain active ingredients including alpha or beta hydroxy acids; home microdermabrasion kits; or mushroom or pumpkin enzymes. Masks, preferably with a clay base, are good for women with oily or acne-prone skin. Apply peels or masks at night, either bimonthly or monthly (see the Appendix for specific brands).

- **Take care of your cosmetics.** If we see one more woman tossing her makeup kit into the back of her roasting-hot car, we're going to make a citizen's arrest. If you abuse your cosmetics, they're going to abuse you right back. Makeup can be a haven for bacteria, so you need to take precautions. Keep your makeup out of heat and sunlight, which can ruin the antibacterials it contains. Make sure the person at the makeup counter wipes container openings before you use the product, so you don't get other customers' souvenirs. And if your foundation, concealer, blush, or other product changes color or smells funny, get rid of it.

- **Be careful with cosmeceuticals.** These are cosmetics with additives such as vitamins or alpha hydroxy acids that have effects similar to pharmaceutical products. Because they are not regulated as drugs, they are subject to misuse. Rather than do it yourself, talk to an aesthetician or dermatologist about cosmeceuticals to make sure they're safe and effective for you.

- **Spend a little on your makeup kit and tools.** We're always trying to find ways to make beauty affordable to every reader, but in some areas, it's possible to be penny-wise and pound-foolish. If you're going to spend money, spend it on the stuff that's next to your skin every day. Shop around, but don't be reluctant to invest in good-quality cosmetics, skin-care products, and tools. Brushes especially should last for years, and the quality of your makeup will go a long way toward ensuring that your skin remains healthy and looking like a million bucks for a long time.

- **In assembling your makeup kit, there are no off-the-rack decisions.** Everything depends on your skin type, complexion,

BEAUTY PEARLS

A great way to keep unruly brows in place is to use clear mascara or a little bit of Vaseline on a clean soft bristle toothbrush and gently brush through your brows. If you've applied too much, you can use the toothbrush to comb through the brow to remove any excess product. Keep in mind that a little goes a long way. Also, if you've overplucked your brows, a great way to temporarily disguise the problem is to apply light strokes of any eyeliner or eye shadow that's a shade lighter than your hair color. Remember to blend with a brow brush or toothbrush to keep your brows looking natural and no one will even notice you've overplucked!

—Anastasia Soare, "The Definitive Eyebrow Expert"

age, race, and skin condition. The best way to start is by consulting with a professional makeup artist and working together to make a shopping list. The basics you've got to have are these: foundation, blush, translucent powder, concealer, lip gloss, lip liner, eye shadow, eyeliner, and mascara. As for specifics—mineral versus liquid makeup, for example—those are questions for your consultant.

• **Practice and learn.** You're not going to be a makeup Matisse overnight. It takes practice. Read books, talk to makeup artists, and try new techniques.

Find your own style. What works for another woman might not work for you. "I've learned to appreciate idiosyncrasy. The fact is, there is really no such thing as 'normal,' " said the late celebrity makeup artist Kevin Aucoin. "Everybody's different, and that is the essence of personal beauty. To forgive yourself your differences and cherish them instead is incredibly liberating. Appreciating individuality is one of the great things about makeup."

Fredericke Grillitz, founder of IQ Beauty, has a refreshingly similar view. Famous for her "light infused" cosmetics, she says, "Less is more. The moment you pass age thirty-five, you should rethink the makeup routine you have had since you were a teenager. You should minimize it—take things away. Do less, and bring out your natural beauty. This is all about enhancing, not hiding. First you need the right product, and then you need to know how to use it."

Sense About Scents

Coco Chanel said, "A woman who doesn't wear perfume has no future." She also called it the unseen, unforgettable, ultimate accessory of fashion. Fragrance is the most personal of beauty adornments, yet it's the one with the most power to enchant from a distance. Before you enter a room and after you leave it, your perfume can be present, announcing or lingering, reminding others of you. Since our sense of smell is powerfully linked to the limbic system of the brain, held to be the home of emotion, fragrance has intense power to shape others' perceptions of you.

There is no "right" perfume for any woman. It's as personal as makeup and jewelry (which we'll get to) and should be equal parts of your personality and the persona you'd like to take on when you dress to the nines for an elegant night out.

Perfume is a complex, three-layered blend of natural botanical and other fragrances, and it's designed to evolve and change over time as it evaporates and your body heat activates certain elements. Thus, what begins with a note of lemon or jasmine will bloom from morning to night into a deeper floral scent and then blend into a deeper tone of sandalwood or musk. A true perfume (as opposed to an eau de toilette) is practically alive and should reflect your character and your sensuality.

Take your time with fragrance, and shop carefully. Test and retest until you find something that speaks to you, and then wear it for a full day before you make your final choice. When you've identified your personal fragrance, use it with discretion. Don't spray it into your hair or on your jewelry (it can damage hair follicles and damage or dull precious metals), and don't rub it into your skin (you could develop a rash). Instead, lightly pat it and let it dry. Subtle fragrances that insinuate themselves into people's senses are the secret behind the magic of perfume. The sense of smell plays a large role in attraction.

One warning: make sure the perfume you select is having the desired effect on those around you. Overpowering perfume is a big turnoff—and some people are allergic.

Bring On the Bling

"Jewelry is a language all its own," says Janice Stevenson, a New York jewelry designer. In our interview, she discussed the evolution and meaning of jewelry from the Stone Age to the present: "Throughout history, we have adorned our bodies with jewelry as talisman or decoration, at our pulse points or against our skin. Jewelry and the relationship with the wearer has inspired artists to create beautiful personal objects worn to ward off evil spirits, celebrate a rite of passage, or simply dazzle the eye. It is infused with rich cultural and personal meanings that express our emotions, heritages, personalities, and moods."

We don rings, necklaces, bracelets, earrings, nail jewels, pins, hair ornaments, anklets, and even fashion eyeglasses and watches to attract attention to a favorite body part, set off our skin color, enhance our overall allure, or make us feel good. Evolution, cultural conditioning, and mass marketing have encouraged us to covet shiny objects (hence our strong attractions to expensive cars and other objects that reflect light).

What kinds of jewelry produce that goddess appeal? That's another personal issue; we all have shapes, colors, stones, or metals that sing to our senses. Wear what speaks to you, whether it's costly designer pieces or inexpensive folk jewelry. The rule of thumb for wearing jewelry is, again, that less is usually more.

Stevenson asserts that selecting and wearing jewelry with which you feel a personal connection can enhance your self-esteem. "Jewelry is often worn to honor a past, such as something inherited from a mother or grandmother," she says. "By giving you a foundation of history, it provides an incredible confidence boost." Stevenson was quick to point out that jewelry is not only for the wealthy crowd. In today's world, one can find inexpensive pieces that complement any outfit and announce your originality. Vintage stores, eBay, and estate sales are excellent places to start looking.

Adorning Your Artwork

We're going to leave specific advice about clothing to fashion designers and wardrobe consultants. The funny thing is, we are joined at the brain when it comes to style. We routinely show up at each other's home wearing the same or very similar clothing. We rolled on the floor the other day when we both walked into a room carrying virtually the same brand-new Banana Republic handbag.

Solely from a physician's perspective, then, here's what we can say about clothing. Just as is the case with physical features, people respond positively to symmetry and averageness in attire. By average, we don't mean dull, but something that meets society's expectations. If you're a fifty-year-old corporate executive, for instance, people are most likely to respond positively to you if you're dressed in a beautifully tailored suit, not jeans and a tank top. Examples of symmetry include matching earrings and one half of an outfit complementing the other, such as a silk blouse matched with finely cut slacks.

On top of this basic formula, our advice is to be surprising. Think what a fabulous crimson scarf can do to set off a steel-gray power suit, or the effect a lustrous string of pearls has on a cashmere sweater. Accessorize with class, but be bold. Conform to society's average, and then defy it slightly. Both men and women respond to variety and a bit of spice. Be a woman in a way that suits you: soft and classic, bold and brassy, young and athletic—whatever works. Accentuate your best features. Wear skirts if you have great legs; wear a belt to show off your waist; and nothing gets attention like a plunging neckline worn by the right person to the right place. That's innate and evolving beauty in action.

Here's what Meg Freeman, a wardrobe stylist for editorial and commercial print and film, has to say about style: "There's a difference between fashion and style. Fashion is a mode that fits a specific time. Style relates to knowing yourself. There's nothing beautiful about a woman wearing what's in fashion if it doesn't fit her shape. Real beauty includes a sense of discrimination and ownership—a sense of someone's inner self finding outward expression in the presentation of her clothes, her hair and makeup, and her manner."

We couldn't have said it better. Now let's go on to the last leg of the Beauty-Brain Loop, your environment.

Beauty Bullets

- Outer beauty reveals the state of your inner beauty and health.

- It's very OK to want to look beautiful.

- Obsessing over perceived flaws in one's appearance is a sign of body dysmorphic disorder.

- Your skin is your body's canvas.

- Number one skin health tip: stay out of the sun!

- Optimal nails and hair demand regular care by professionals.

- Dental health affects both your attractiveness and your overall health.

- Tooth whitening or veneers can be an easy path to a winning smile and better self-esteem.

- Makeup, fragrance, and jewelry are highly personal beauty choices that you should take your time making, relying on professional advice.

- Your beauty regimen should evolve as the years pass.

BEAUTY AND THE BRAIN Rx

Making Changes

Dr. Debra: *Make a list of your three top cosmetic priorities (fat reduction, skin improvement, wrinkle reduction, acne treatment, teeth bleaching, hair coloring, etc.). Create a budget and a time line for accomplishing them. Gone are the days when women waited until a certain age to enhance and improve their looks with some judicious cosmetic surgery. Today's women need a life plan for beauty maintenance that includes small cosmetic replacements and enhancements along the road, ranging from as early as the teens to seventy and beyond. Take your list to your facialist, hairdresser, dentist, and dermatologist, as appropriate, and get an honest assessment of the risks, benefits, and costs of each procedure.*

Dr. Eva: *Make sure that your pursuit of beauty is coming from a healthy place. These enhancements should make you look and feel better. Signs that your beauty regimen is becoming unhealthy include the following: spending money you don't have; being repeatedly dissatisfied with treatments; feeling that no matter what you do, you will never look good enough; spending excessive time on grooming; and allowing your appearance to negatively affect your work or relationships.*

7

Environment: Living in the World You Make

People are more apt to believe you and like you when you know you look fine. And when the world approves, self-respect is just a little easier.

—Estée Lauder

KATRINA IS AN operatic soprano in her late thirties with a big mane of blonde hair and a curvy figure. Despite her physical attributes, for years, no one noticed her. She didn't let herself be noticed, in part because she was hiding the truth that her marriage was emotionally diseased. She felt embarrassed about who she was. When the marriage finally ended, Katrina found a surprise: the woman she'd always thought she could be.

One day as she was walking into a hotel with some coworkers, for the first time in her life, a man driving by stopped his car and stuck his head out the window to tell her she was beautiful. She hadn't lost weight or changed anything about how she looked, but she had a new swagger, a strut that reflected her stronger self-esteem. It literally stopped traffic.

"I'll never forget that moment, but the beauty came from the inside out," she said. "I actually felt free and beautifully vulnerable. I remember looking in the mirror that day, thinking I was beautiful and who was that girl? Where had she been? After the one who is supposed to love you hasn't given you a compliment in years, it's hurtful, and when a stranger says it . . . it still brings tears to my eyes."

COLLECTING YOUR REWARD

That's a splendid example of the environment responding to inner beauty. Environment is the final stage in the Beauty-Brain Loop. We're referring not to the save-the-redwoods kind of environment (though that's important, too) but to the world around you. Everything outside of your body and mind is your environment: your home, career, social circle, pastimes, community, and relationships.

Environment is a unique stage of the loop in that its rewards are often instantaneous. When you activate the power of the loop by initiating change in any of the other stages, you might not see the results as quickly. For example, if you change your outer beauty by getting a hip new hairstyle, your inner beauty will improve. Certainly, if you start a workout and nutrition program, it can take weeks before you see big improvements in your energy level and the fit of your clothes. The environment, however, gives you feedback, positive or negative, right away. Get that hip new hairstyle, and you'll get compliments the very next day.

Another distinction of the environment is that it's not passive. If you dress like a bag lady or are habitually gloomy, it's highly improbable that someone will come up to you and declare, "Heavens, you look smashing!" Positive feedback from your environment has to be earned. It's the payoff window of the loop, where all the

BEAUTY BUDDIES

Mary Mayotte, nationally known communications coach, founder of Mary Mayotte + Associates, and head coach of the Speech Fitness Institute, speechfitness.com

I've had so many Beauty Buddies—as a communications/media and executive coach for fifteen years, I consider my clients some of my best beauty resources. I enjoy mixing their expertise with simple beauty "pleasures" that we share when celebrating birthdays and our successes.

As a TV personality, Ford model, and spokesperson in the beauty business for twenty years prior to my coaching career, I have worked from every angle on new product launches for all of the major cosmetics brands from Clinique and Oil of Olay to Cover Girl and L'Oréal. I have been so fortunate to have coached celebrity spokespersons like Nikki Taylor, Christie Brinkley, and Faith Hill and celebrity hair and makeup artists from Rita Hazan, Danilo, Laura Mercier, and Susan Sterling of Chanel. Sharing fun with them makes work a pleasure. I've gotten to know so many of my clients personally over the years that they've become my friends and staunchest supporters. I derive a lot of my passion for this business from them and get my best fashion and beauty tips as well.

Just a few of the people who have inspired me:

- *Charla Krupp, fashion and beauty editor and author of* **How Not to Look Old:** *Charla always offers great tips on how to shop and what to wear to be your best and be completely appropriate at any age.*

- *Ricky Lauren:* I'm lucky to be in a business where I'm inspired all the time by special people like Ricky Lauren, Ralph's wife. Sustained by her family life, she's a beautiful and talented psychologist and author, and she is

(continued)

so wonderful at entertaining. She's a fabulous, elegant, and graceful woman whom I completely admire.

• **My thirty-eight fantastic hosts from Home Shopping Network:** They know all there is to know about looking and feeling beautiful in mind, body, and soul. These women are awe inspiring and quite beautiful inside and out.

I think the real long-distance runners, if you will, help to create beauty everywhere with their innate and generous spirits. I'm blessed that women (and men) like these are my Beauty Buddies par excellence! I'm so lucky to be working with them.

self-awareness and diligent work pay off. That's what gives environment its power. At the end of the day, when you have done the cognitive heavy lifting to become more optimistic, ratcheted up your fruit and vegetable intake, and forked over a king's ransom on stylish new attire, you enjoy the compliments. You like to be recognized as a new and improved woman. Your environment gives you that feedback and encourages you to keep making positive changes.

Of course, you can also set the loop in motion by making changes in your environment that ignite changes elsewhere. Beautifying your home and creating spaces for peaceful meditation, quiet time with loved ones, or your beauty regimen can work wonders. Going on vacations, especially to places that you've always dreamed of visiting, can fortify the old self-esteem and optimism. Gathering friends together for long dinners, nights out, or just wandering conversation is a fantastic way to transform your environment. All of these actions make you feel more positive, reduce stress, and motivate you to institute more changes for the better.

A "Sex and the City" World

We all know a few people who appear to inhabit a world right out of a Hollywood soundstage. For them, life seems to unroll the red carpet. They have glorious careers that pay them a small fortune. They have astonishing homes and gleaming luxury cars. They have storybook relationships, and if they have children, the kids are well scrubbed and faultlessly mannered. Everything seems to go swimmingly for these people. They meet all the right people, make all the right moves, and reap the rewards. Matter of fact, their lives are so perfect that no Hollywood scriptwriter would concoct such a story.

Nobody lives in a cinematic nirvana where doing everything right gives you a guarantee of being beautiful and adored. We live in a place that's more like "Sex and the City," in which we're charming and debonair one day, and then the next, we topple off a fashion-show runway in front of hundreds, betrayed by a pair of wretched four-inch heels. In the spirit of Carrie and Samantha, we do the best we can, but the world is largely what we make of it. In the "Sex and the City" world, people fall down, mess up, and get their hearts broken. Regardless, they forge ahead from day to day. In all probability, you're more like Carrie and the gang. So, what's the secret of the people who seem to have perfect lives?

There is no secret. People for whom the world is an oyster are maximizing the power of the Beauty-Brain Loop. They look as beautiful as their genes will allow. They're in supreme shape and obvious excellent health. They dress immaculately. They're positive and confident and wise and flirtatious and witty. They're unfailingly generous, gracious, and ethical. In short, they're giving their environment the richest possible input as fodder. In return, the environment lavishes them with rewards. They're attractive and magnetic in the ways we talked about earlier. The best people and the rarest opportunities come their way regularly. Nobody is perfect, but they do the best they can. That's all any of us can do.

Here's an illustration of how the loop works in your environment:

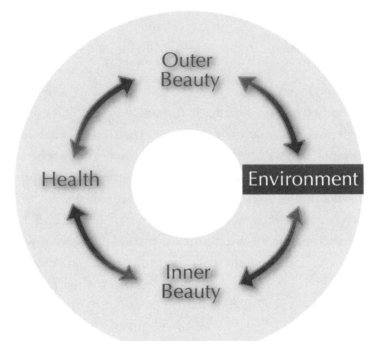

Each step reinforces the other. New confidence leads to new possibilities, which further invigorate your self-esteem and inner beauty. That's a formula for loving not only yourself but also your entire life. Even more than that, it's a way to create the world in which you want to dwell.

✍ BEAUTY STORY: "HEATHER"

Heather, forty-six, came to see Debra to explore some cosmetic "refreshing." She had a "turkey neck" and under-eye circles, both common. After a consultation, she decided to think it over for a while. About six months later, she returned to Debra's office and revealed that just after her last visit, she had learned she had breast cancer. She had undergone moderate chemotherapy and was in remission. Now she wanted to go ahead with the cosmetic procedures she and Debra had discussed. She wanted to tell the world, and herself, that she was healthy and feeling good. So, she had the cosmetic work that she had delayed before: Botox and Thermage.

Eva: I think Heather came at this from a really healthy perspective. She no longer looked healthy when you saw her the second time; she looked as if she'd been through the mill, and she had. Chemotherapy can be brutal on the body, so she wanted to prove to herself and her environment that she had come back.

Debra: When I first saw her, before she knew about her cancer, she struck me as a very together woman who wanted advice about making some small improvements in her appearance. When she approached me after her cancer therapy, I could see that she still had the same attitude. This was not a cure-all or a denial. It was a way of saying, "OK, I'm moving on."

REFLECTIONS OF YOU

There is a biological basis to the way people respond to you, for better or worse. The brain has what are called "mirror neurons," areas that read and reflect the facial expressions, breathing, and muscle activity of other people in close proximity. These mirror neurons stimulate the brain to mimic the emotional state of the person being observed. So, it figures that we want to be around people who are self-assured, positive, funny, and sexy. Our brains want the chemical rewards that come with having those same emotions ourselves.

Remember the research showing that beautiful people earn more money and get breaks from the legal system? Mirror neurons are a big part of the reason why. Beautiful people stimulate our innate sense of beauty and make us feel good about ourselves. That's why we go out of our way to do things for them. This applies not just to physical beauty but to self-esteem and personality as well. If you are average looking but overpoweringly positive and enthusiastic, you'll have the same effect on people. In fact, while physical beauty might make a better first impression, an ordinary-looking women with a brilliant mind and a positive personality will get more rewards from the environment than a gorgeous woman who is neurotic and unpleasant. Inner beauty can move mountains.

Women appear to have more mirror neurons than men. This makes sense, as we evolved being the primary caretakers for babies and children. We needed nonverbal ways to figure out what our charges were trying to tell us. Our abundance of mirror neurons makes us more empathetic, and we derive more emotional benefits from spending time with positive people. By the same token, it also means we're walking emotion detectors and are just as susceptible to catching negative emotions. Women sometimes anticipate and match the emotions—and their physical effects—of the person they're with. Emotions are contagious, and if you're spending time with someone whose signals are gloomy or irate, you can become emotionally "infected." It's also been suggested that because of estrogen, women feel the physical effects of intuition—the knot in the stomach, blushing, and so on—more strongly than men. The "gut feeling" really hits like a punch in the solar plexus.

Because we want to be around people who exhibit the emotions we'd like to exhibit, people with great inner beauty make us feel better. On the other end are those who make us want

---

BEAUTY BOOSTERS

Practical things you can do now to be more beautiful

Eva: One sure thing you can do to become more beautiful and appealing to others is to learn to become a better listener. Many of us are poor listeners; while another person is speaking, we spend much of our time waiting for our turn, rehearsing what we're going to say. This behavior is obvious to other people, and it makes us less attractive to them. It's natural for people to want to feel that what they have to say is important to the hearer.

Try to become a more active listener. You can take a cue from Native American traditions, which honor these four principles:

- *Silence: Be completely quiet and attentive when another person is speaking.*

- *Spontaneity: Don't worry about what you will say when the person is done speaking. It will take care of itself. Active listening will guide you to a response.*

- *Honesty: Be honest and caring in your response, no matter what has been said.*

- *Gratitude: Be thankful that the other person has chosen to share part of his or her story with you. Remember that nobody has to trust you as a listener.*

to run in the other direction. They are the ones with such low self-esteem that they can't stop talking about themselves. They never pause to listen. They seem to suck the room dry of energy, and that's not an illusion. Psychologist Matthew Lieberman has observed that emotions tend to flow from the most powerful person in the room to others.

Bottom line, you can attract or repel others based solely on your inner life. The decisive factor is how you live your life all the time. Caring for your body and mind, empowering yourself, and setting and reaching goals all contribute to a permanent state of contagious beauty. You also need to surround yourself with positive people. They will lift you up and make you more beautiful inside and out.

Environment and the Loop

Nowhere will you experience the effects of changes in your inner beauty, health, or outer beauty more starkly than in your environment. The environment is the strongest reward system in the Beauty-Brain Loop. Sure, after you've spent a year hitting the treadmill and pumping iron, it's nice to look in the mirror and see a slender figure, and it feels good to visit your doctor and learn that your blood pressure and cholesterol are perfect. Still, nothing beats a friend at a party saying, "Wow, you look awesome!"

The environment is like wet sand: everything you do makes an impression. Your self-esteem, the way you dress, how you handle stress, the foods you eat—it all affects how your environment reacts to you. Most of the time, the reaction is subtle; if you constantly appear stressed, people will form a more negative opinion of you without saying a word about it. Nevertheless, over time, it all adds up. More important, the environmental reaction shapes the other stages of the loop. Social approval lifts your self-confidence and prompts you to become even more fit. Get a promotion at work and you'll start dressing more elegantly. And the feedback continues. Your environment is reactive, and it can catalyze powerful responses in the rest of your life.

THE SCIENCE OF BEING COOL

People are social beings. We seek out the company of others. That's why when Saturday night rolls around and you go out with friends even when you'd rather stay home and watch "Gilmore Girls" Season One on DVD, you feel better. You know that if you'd stayed in alone, you would have felt lazy, bored, and bummed out. Being with other people makes us feel charged up and complete, and our inner beauty can have the same effect on others.

Can someone develop charisma? Scientists are actually starting to research this, trying to figure out what makes some people fountains of magnetism while others are buzz killers. Ronald Riggio, Ph.D., a psychology professor at Claremont McKenna College, in California, believes that charm has three key components: expressivity, sensitivity, and control. In his view, a charming individual not only is able to bring out feelings in others but also can read and respond to the emotions of others instantly. Another researcher, Frank Bernieri, Ph.D., of Oregon State University, proposes that a major factor in charisma is *synchrony*, the ability to compel the person with whom you're communicating to unconsciously match your gestures and physicality. Still other researchers approach charisma from the other side and argue that the ability to subtly mimic a listener, from breathing rhythm to gestures, creates a connection. No one knows if charisma

---

BEAUTY PEARLS

A woman is most beautiful when she is open, present, conscious of her feelings and her behavior, and connected to the world around her. One piece of advice to help women become their most beautiful: make kindness your religion. The better you feel about the things you do, the better you'll feel about the way you look.

—*Valerie Monroe, beauty director, O, The Oprah Magazine*

---

is inborn or learned from situations, but one thing is certain: cultivating social adeptness and the ability to listen actively and be completely with the person to whom you're speaking is very possible and yields personal dividends.

"ACT YOUR AGE" ISN'T JUST FOR TEENAGERS

Sad to say, no amount of charm will rescue you from being ridiculous. We're talking about the woman who is—and let's be generous here—well beyond the age of arriving at a social event wearing low-rise jeans, a belly chain, and a see-through top with a black bra. Even if you have the body for this, it's just not appropriate when you're fifty. It doesn't matter what environment you're in, how fit you are, or how young your date is. Simply. Not. Apropos. End of story.

Part of turning your environment into your oyster and remaking your world the way you want it is being age-appropriate and classy. Dressing twenty years too young doesn't suggest, "I'm a free spirit who plays by her own rules." It screams, "I'm desper-

---

BEAUTY BUSTERS

Beauty myths debunked while you wait

Myth: People in healthy relationships don't argue or fight.

Fact: If you know two people who supposedly "never fight," one of three things is going on with their relationship. Either they're lying through their teeth, they don't communicate at all, or one is a doormat for the other. There is absolutely nothing wrong with healthy disagreement in a romantic relationship or friendship; it shows that both people are adults with their own minds and opinions. Occasional arguments can clear the air and release tension. Just follow these rules for healthy fighting:

- *Rule number one: No hitting below the belt. Don't get personal or dredge up past offenses. Then you're moving from making a point to fighting just to injure.*

- *Rule number two: No grabbing and holding. Not every fight has to have a winner. Sometimes, it's OK to agree to disagree and move on.*

- *Rule number three: No going to bed mad. Always make up (in whatever way is most fun) before you end the day or say good-bye. Grudges turn into anger and resentment. Try not to hold a grudge. Refocus as soon as you can on the positives in the relationship and work together to find solutions.*

---

ate for attention!" Think about some famous women well into middle age who are always elegant, sexy, and gorgeous: Susan Sarandon, Sela Ward, Kim Cattrall, Jane Seymour, Diane Lane, Rene Russo, Sigourney Weaver, Sharon Stone. Think they would show up for the Oscars in something that looked as if it belonged on someone half their age? Not in a million years.

You can look sultry and classy and still look your age. If you're at middle age, one of the advantages is that you can get away with classic, old-time Hollywood looks that a younger woman can't pull off. Your confidence and intelligence just enhance that stunning effect. Part of making the most of your environment is making a perfect package of style, beauty, and experience.

BEAUTY, BEAUTY EVERYWHERE

When you make yourself more beautiful, you're doing much more than creating a better reflection. You're adding to the sum total of beauty in the world, and that's marvelous. We've spoken about how important it is, as you try to develop your evolving beauty, to train yourself to develop an artist's eye and see more beauty around you. That is a terrific way to enhance your self-esteem and be more positive about life, but there are two ways you can extend this even further: by helping others to see more beauty around them and by creating beauty yourself.

When you learn to see something ravishing in the cracked glazing of an antique pot or the riot of an untended garden, it's as if you're looking through the eyes of an artist or a photographer. Well, why not help someone else acquire that same gift? Once you have begun to retrain your perceptions, introduce a friend to the notion. Go out on the town together and help your companion spot all the signs of subtle beauty that most of us never notice: detailing on old buildings, quirky signs on shops, the spirited music from passing cars. Beauty is everywhere, and when you teach another woman to start recognizing it, you're helping her to recognize that society's standard of beauty is only one way to be beautiful. You add one more voice to the chorus of people claiming that true beauty is about who and what you are, not just how you look.

And why not go all the way and create your own beauty? Instead of being an interested observer, add to the beauty that others can see. You do this when you bring out your own inner and outer beauty, but why stop there? Express your own natural gifts by bringing more beauty into your world. This means different things for different women. It could be giving a friend a makeover or helping turn a vacant lot in the neighborhood into a community garden. Be creative, and remember that beauty isn't just visual but includes sounds, smells, and textures as well. If you're a spectacular cook, make dishes that fill the air with delicious smells. Create wind chimes that turn breezes into song.

You have limitless ways to create beauty that others can appreciate. When you teach your eyes to recognize beauty everywhere you look, share that gift with a girlfriend or family member, and then become a participant in the beauty parade by making your own, you're truly becoming an artist, with your environment as your canvas.

BE A RELATIONSHIP CHEF

In the end, our truest expression of beauty in the environment is in our relationships. With apologies to John Donne, no woman is an island; you are not only the person that you see in the mirror but also the perceptions of everyone who comes into contact with you. You should be using your wisdom, love, and compassion to improve the depth and quality of every relationship in your life. All relationships take work, but what endeavor is more worthwhile?

The two of us have been lucky enough to be in each other's lives for more than a quarter of a century now. With love, joy, and friendship, we've seen each other through a lot of highs and lows, from health issues to the loss of parents. We leaned on each other in school, studying holed up at Harvard's Countway Library every night until closing. In our sparse free time, we would host "theme" dinners for our friends, dressing up in all kinds of costumes that went with the theme (for Japanese night, it was kimonos). When we got married, synchronicity hit again: our ceremonies were within six months of each other. Debra's mother made us both beautiful crystal veil headbands. Six months apart, again, our daughters were born.

Relationships are like fine cuisine: you get out of them exactly what you put in. Make the most of your self-knowledge and your giving spirit and become a chef in your personal life. As we age, the shallow rewards of life that we craved when we were younger tend to become less substantial. After all, been there, done that.

Women appear to be genetically built for intimate friendships with each other. Close relationships between women seem to make us healthier and happier and even to enhance the survival of the species. Being in close contact sets off the brain's hormonal reward circuitry, making it a balm to spend time with the girls at the beauty salon or talking over a cup of tea. Even more intriguing, Chris Dunkel Schetter, a UCLA psychologist, has found that women who are the most social tend to have healthier babies. In 2000, she interviewed 247 pregnant women and discovered that the more support and nurturing the women received from family and friends, the higher their babies' birth weights were. Being together really is good for us.

As we become more complete women, expressing all our levels of beauty, we become more generous. We don't need artificial expressions of admiration to make us feel upbeat about ourselves. We need people—people we love, admire, and cherish; people who challenge us, make us better, and love us no matter what we did the day before. Women draw strength from relationships, from shared time and histories. As time moves along, our relationships become our true works of art.

So, the second-best advice we can give you (we'll get to the best in a moment) about your environment is simple: look to your relationships with everyone in your life. Family takes first priority, of course, but don't stop there. Friends, colleagues, community servants, and even idle acquaintances can all add something to your life. So, add something to theirs. With strong inner beauty, you have love to share, so share it. Communicate. Express your gratitude. Forgive. Remind the people in your life how much they mean to you. Also seek out new relationships with people who bring something new to your life, a fresh point of view or a life story you've never heard before. Make time and space for people—to listen, to share, and simply to be.

THE MEDIA DETOX

We've spent a fair amount of ink in this book denouncing the media's 24-7 beauty machine and how it brainwashes us into hating our bodies and wanting to be perfect. Alas, nothing we say here is going to turn off the envy machine that fires up when you see a twenty-year-old coed stroll by wearing a bikini top and a prayer. That's why we herewith introduce the Beauty Prescription Media Detox.

This detox plan is straightforward: Take a break from the distorted images on television as well as from the supermarket magazines, the self-help books that make you feel broken, and the gossip sessions dedicated to trashing other women. Switch to magazines and shows that embrace positive messages that promote health for your body and mind. You don't have to cut yourself off from all media; just try to take it all less seriously. Don't believe everything you see or hear. Remember, models and actresses are usually airbrushed or Photoshopped, and they're real people just like you, with real strengths and weaknesses.

When you give less weight to these images, you liberate yourself to take on a more positive outlook, worry less about how other women look, and spend more time in productive pursuits with your body and mind.

THIS MAGIC MOMENT

Oh yes, that best piece of advice we can give you about the environment? It's this: *Be in the moment.*

We're not always good at the moment. We're very busy, you see. We have important places to go, things to get done. We have lists. But in the rush to be somewhere, we can forget to be where we are. So, stop. Just stop and listen. Look around. Remember that in all of time, there will never be another moment like the one you're experiencing right now, as you sit reading this book. Ever. Notice the sounds, sights, and scents around you. Try taking a mental photograph of the moment in all its detail. Before you go to bed, make a mental list of everything that was good about the day. See the mundane and the grand. It's all beautiful, because it's exquisitely rare. It's all a gift.

Beauty Bullets

ᴥ The environment reacts to beauty and contains beauty.

ᴥ The more you do right, the more readily the world falls into place for you.

- You can poison your environment with foolish choices in the other stages of the Beauty-Brain Loop.

- Social grace and charm can be learned.

- Acting your age can be gorgeous, classy, and sexy.

- Try to help others see more beauty around them, and create your own.

- Live in the moment, because each moment is a gift.

BEAUTY AND THE BRAIN Rx

Be an Environmentalist: Clearing the Cobwebs

Dr. Debra: *Organize your beauty environment so it's accessible to you. Make sense of your closet and makeup drawers so you can locate the things you need when you need them. Store your makeup properly so it lasts, remains free of bacteria, and looks good for its lifetime. After all, cosmetics are a substantial investment. Have a skin-care regimen; write it down, and tape it to your mirror. Carve out a beautiful space where you can sit for ten to thirty minutes every day and just listen, watch, and let your mind wander. Take a warm, spa-like bath as often as you can. Create your own "beauty space" in your home, the place you come to feel and become as beautiful and healthy as you can be.*

Dr. Eva: *Do a spring cleaning, not just of your house but also of your mind and your life. Stuff piles up in our lives when we're busy running in ten different directions. Getting things in order simplifies your existence and cre-*

(continued)

ates room for positive transformation to happen. When you feel as if you can barely breathe under your layers of obligation, emotional baggage, and physical clutter, get down to some cleaning. It is wondrous what clearing out what you don't need anymore can do for your spirits. Those old grudges and resentments from past relationships? Throw them out with the memorabilia from your college summer vacations and your ancient computer. Life is about not just what we keep but also what we have the courage to let go.

Beautiful for Life

8

Staying Beautiful Through the Years

*Character contributes to beauty. It fortifies a woman
as her youth fades. A mode of conduct, a standard of
courage, discipline, fortitude, and integrity can do a
great deal to make a woman beautiful.*

—Jacqueline Bisset

A 2005 SURVEY BY *Allure* magazine called "The Allure of
Beauty Study" produced some results that were surprisingly
refreshing. The survey of more than seventeen hundred men and
women revealed that Americans consider women over age fifty to
be just as beautiful as women under thirty. What raised perfectly
tweezed eyebrows all over the country was the fact that when
asked to name the most beautiful woman alive, the respondents
primarily named women between the ages of fifty and seventy.
The most commonly chosen women included perennial beauty
Sophia Loren but also Oprah Winfrey and Meryl Streep.

As much as we, other health-care professionals, and soci-
ologists might fret over the effects of our reputedly beauty-
worshipping, inadequacy-fueling culture, this is pretty hopeful

stuff. If men and women are seeing past the plastic fantastic of celebrity coverage and photo retouching to the inner beauty in women of all ages, then maybe we're not headed for a desperate, insecure future. Perhaps we can look forward to a time when "real" women—crow's-feet, gray hair, and all—grace the covers of our most popular magazines and are considered sexy.

 ## BEAUTY BUDDIES

Diane Ranger, inventor of mineral makeup and founder of Colorescience, and Cynthia Rowland, creator of Facial Magic

What do these two beauty pioneers have in common? Aside from their friendship, a genuine admiration for each other's beauty wisdom. "Cynthia has taught me the importance of facial exercises," says Diane. "As with the body, the exercise gets the oxygen flowing and helps tighten sagging skin."

"Diane Ranger is more than a Beauty Buddy; she's a living doll!" says Cynthia. "A mutual friend from Toronto insisted that we meet because she knew we were like-minded when it came to beauty. Diane's mineral makeup line, Colorescience, was very interesting to me because I like natural remedies rather than synthetic chemicals. I wanted to know all about her line so that my face would look sensational."

The two began spending beauty time together after meeting for lunch and exchanging products: Colorescience mineral makeup from Diane, a copy of Cynthia's facial exercise instructional video. This led to a spa date; lunch at a Long Beach, California, Lebanese restaurant; and a continuing series of get-togethers focused on beauty and having fun. They also learned how to attract a crowd.

"Once when we were facial exercising in the Montage [a Laguna Beach, California, hotel] restroom, we were drawing quite a crowd of inter-

ested women and that was somehow reported to the management," says
Cynthia. "The 'bathroom police' arrived wanting to know exactly what was
going on! Diane has the most wonderful gift of gab and she talked our way
out of the bathroom."

Both ladies cherish the beauty time they share. "Physically it really gets
my face in shape and gets the oxygen flowing," Diane says. "Mentally it is
great female bonding with another woman on a similar mission."

Cynthia agrees: "The time we share is precious. Here we are two businesswomen who work long hours, travel frequently, and much is required
of us. When we're enjoying the Montage, the spa, or just a salad somewhere, nothing else matters to us! We can relax and enjoy our stimulating conversations, which seem to charge our batteries until we're together
again."

Asked what about the other is beautiful to them, both Diane and Cynthia were emphatic. "Cynthia has a big heart and she lets it lead her life
decisions," says Diane. Cynthia's response? "I think women can take a
lesson from Diane. She is the ultimate steel magnolia and an accessible
friend. She is just so willing and flexible towards life . . . that makes her fun!
She wants to make life exciting and happening for women. Life is not about
competition; rather, it is really meaningful when you help another person in
words and in deeds."

Now, that's not an excuse to binge on Ben & Jerry's. You'll
notice that the three beauties named in the survey are women
who take exquisite care of their bodies and minds. Part of the
reason they're beautiful is that they respect themselves enough
to care for their skin, hair, and health over a lifetime, as well as
cultivating charisma and passion for a life that they clearly love.

It's not OK to look at the results of the *Allure* survey and say, "Yes, I get a free pass!" No matter how old you are, no matter how genetically gifted you may be, if you want to be thought of as a timeless beauty, you've got to take care of yourself—starting now. There are no shortcuts or free passes.

THE REALITY OF MONEY

As we leave talk of the Beauty-Brain Loop behind for now, a serious question arises: How the heck do we do all these things for the rest of our lives? We hear some variation on that question all the time from women who are exceedingly accomplished and dreadfully busy. They're moms, owners of companies, award-winning artists, fellow physicians, or athletes—sometimes several of the above at once—and every one of them is trying to balance the needs to look as good as possible with the need to just survive the day. You know that look you used to get from your mother when you said or did something that really made her mad? Suggest to today's female high achiever that she needs to spend more time on her beauty regimen and you'll get the same icy stare.

Deep down, though, every one of us knows that beauty—the inner or outer variety—isn't free. It costs time and effort and money. And we know that if we neglect it now, we'll pay for it later in desperate cosmetic surgeries, tearful regrets, and damaged self-esteem. But we've also got schedules to keep and miles to go before we head to the spa for a facial. What we need is a plan . . . a plan to which we can stick for life. As luck would have it, that's precisely what awaits you in this chapter.

Another component in play is, of course, money. Premium beauty products can be obscenely expensive, and since insurance companies usually consider cosmetic surgery to be elective, it can

---

BEAUTY STORY: "JULIE"

Julie, a twenty-three-year-old graduate student in management, came to Debra interested in lip enhancement. This is a popular procedure with young women, because many models have enlarged lips. Julie specified that she wanted lips that were out of proportion with her face. Debra counseled her that overly large lips would not enhance her appearance and in the end gave Julie Restylane injections to plump up her lips but kept them in proportion to her facial features.

Debra: *I wish I could say I'm surprised at these beautiful young women who come to me so unhappy with their lips, but I see it so much that I know what they're going to say as soon as they walk in. I was named by a local entertainment magazine as the dermatologist to go to for fillers and lip injections, so women who want "lips like the stars" often seek me out.*

Eva: *It's unfortunate that so many young ladies who are stunning aren't pleased with their appearance. They can be swayed by the media images they see and they think they need to fit a stereotype. Yes, evolution has made men attracted to full lips as a sign of fertility, but it's really the whole package that's important. Obsessing over a flaw or wanting exaggerated features may be a sign of deeper issues.*

---

be completely out of reach for many women. So, that comprehensive plan that you can follow for decades also has to fit into even a moderate budget. In keeping with those confines, we've endeavored to stay firmly in the real world to bring you a Life Beauty Plan that makes good common sense.

This plan features noninvasive treatments for your skin as well as behavioral tips for your mind. After all, we're a dermatologist and a psychiatrist, and we stick to our specialties. Check out the Resources section at the back of the book for recommended books, magazines, and other sources of information that will enhance what we're telling you here. A few things to keep in mind:

- Your needs will change as you age.
- Your beauty budget will increase as you age. The more time that passes, the more Benjamins you're going to hand over to stay looking good.
- Long-term commitment is the key to success.
- This is a generalized plan. Talk to your dermatologist to customize it for your unique needs.

THE BEAUTY PRESCRIPTION LIFE BEAUTY PLAN

The real work of beauty starts in your twenties. In Chapter 6, we gave you our daily skin-care regimen. Here we offer a decade-by-decade review of skin-care procedures that you can have done by a professional—an aesthetician in some cases, but in most cases, a dermatologist.

Note: The costs listed are approximate ranges per treatment; they will change over time and may vary depending on the region of the country in which you live.

Ages Twenty to Thirty

Your hormones may still be balancing. You can have acne due to a possible increase in oil by the sebaceous glands. During this time, you should begin laying the foundation for lifelong beauty by starting some basic skin-care routines. If you have dry skin, put a moisturizer on and use sunscreen daily. You may still have occasional breakouts, and for some women, this is when sun damage will start to appear.

Procedure	Frequency	Cost per treatment
Glycolic acid peel or microdermabrasion	Every 3 months	$150–$200

Ages Thirty to Forty

Here's where you start to pay the price for those days in your twenties baking at the beach competing to see who could get the darkest tan. Sun damage may be settling in, bringing with it fine lines. You may also start to see frown lines becoming more visible, which ironically can make you frown even more. How cruel.

This is when *dynamic* wrinkles can start. These are wrinkles you get from muscular contractions such as smiling or frowning. Botox affects dynamic wrinkles. *Static* wrinkles are caused by sun damage. This period is a major turning point for your skin. Your metabolism starts slowing down, and muscle lines are starting to take form. Your skin is less able to replace its cells, so whereas when you were younger, it took twenty days to replace all your surface skin cells, now it takes forty.

Start getting chemical peels from a professional, doing home peels, and having checks for skin cancers. Melanoma, which can be fatal, is most frequent in women between twenty and forty-five. This is also a time when your stress levels are likely to produce inflammation, wrinkling, and sagging in your skin.

BEAUTY BOOSTERS

Practical things you can do now to be more beautiful

Did you know that about 70 percent of household dust comprises dead skin cells? It's true. You're constantly shedding dead skin to make room for new, healthy skin. However, much of the time, this process isn't fast enough on its own to keep your skin looking its best. That's why as the years go on, the skin can start looking dull from the buildup of dead skin cells. So, give the shedding a little help. Home peels such as Neutrogena Advanced Solutions Facial Peel are a gentle way to start. Made of mushroom proteins, it can be used one to two times a week. For a more active home peel, try Kinerase Instant Radiance Facial Peel. This product is made from lactic and fruit acids. It is delivered on premoistened swabs and applied daily for five days, with an interval of two weeks between peels.

Cortisol-inducing foods such as caffeine and alcohol can also bring on wrinkling, irritation, and inflammation, so it's wise to consume less of them or eschew them completely. Just as your skin is not what it used to be, neither is your liver. Your ability to metabolize toxins will decrease, and the negative effects of caffeine and alcohol will be multiplied.

This is likewise the stage when rosacea tends to develop. The disease has become more common in our society, and the reason for that is unclear. It typically appears as flushing and pink bumps around the mouth and is made worse by hormone fluctuations, stress, exercise, and alcohol. Fortunately, there are some effective treatments for rosacea. If you develop it, you're in good company: Bill Clinton and Princess Diana presumably had it.

Procedure	Frequency	Cost per treatment
Botox for dynamic wrinkles and frown lines (the "11" lines between your brows)	Every 3–6 months	$500–$1,000
Glycolic peels or microderm-abrasion for mild sun damage and dull skin	Monthly	$150–$200
If you have sun damage (hyper-pigmentation, etc.), then intense pulse light (IPL) or photo facial or Fraxel laser	5 times first year, 1–3 times per year thereafter	$400–$600

Ages Forty to Fifty

Now the changes of aging become more visible, especially as you approach menopause. The lady who invented the T-shirt that reads "I'm out of estrogen and I have a gun" was right on the money. Your skin's elasticity is decreasing, and things are starting to sag around the neck and jawline. Dynamic wrinkles are becoming more apparent. Your skin is losing its luster, and sun damage is becoming more visible. Things are changing fast. To keep them as under control as you can, follow as much of this plan as possible.

You're starting to get perimenopausal, when lack of estrogen begins to make the skin look duller and reduces its elasticity. You might start looking more wrinkled and aged. Also, you may have other health challenges and be taking medications, which can contribute to the skin's looking more aged or dull.

This set of circumstances makes it more imposing than ever to be on top of your skin-care ritual. You may even want to make some adaptations to your routine to focus more on your current skin challenges. This is a time to start a regular routine with retinoids. Prescription-strength retinoids such as Retin-A or Renova are the only topicals proven to increase collagen formation and decrease degeneration. In addition, skin cancers—basal cell, squamous cell—start appearing at this age due to years of sun exposure. Start doing a monthly skin exam as you would do a breast exam. Check for anything that feels like a grain of sand because it could be precancerous. Look for shiny pink bumps; those could be basal cells. These cancers are easily treatable if caught early.

Also consider eating more phytoestrogens—nutrients contained in soy, flaxseed, chickpeas, bran, and several other foods. These chemical compounds mimic the body's estrogen and appear to help prevent bone loss as you age. Also, if you're not getting enough exercise, increase your amount of aerobic activity and add strength training to build muscle, boost your metabolism, and add bone mass.

Procedure	Frequency	Cost per treatment
Botox for forehead wrinkles, frown lines, and crow's-feet	Every 3–6 months	$700–$1,500
Fillers—Juvéderm, Perlane, Restylane, Cosmoderm, Cosmoplast, Radiesse, Sculptra—for lines around the mouth and "marionette" lines	1–2 syringes every 6–12 months	$1,000–$4,000
Radio-frequency skin tightening (Thermage)	Every 2 years	$1,300–$6,000

If you have moderate sun damage, IPL treatment	5 times the first year, 2–3 times per year thereafter	$400
If you have severe sun damage, photodynamic therapy	3–4 treatments, repeated every 3–5 years	$800
Fractional laser (Fraxel) treatment	3–5 sessions, 1 every 2 weeks; the results last 5–10 years	$1,200–$2,000

Ages Fifty to Sixty

If you've been taking care of your skin, you should be able to remain in a holding pattern, aside from making some extra effort to counter the normal effects of aging. You might notice that nasolabial lines are starting to run from your nose to your mouth, as well as "marionette" lines from your mouth to your chin. You might also see some sagging in your jowls. During this time, you should be consuming essential fatty acids such as omega-3s, avoiding alcohol and caffeine, and keeping up with exercise and self-exams. Also, consider nonsurgical face-lifts such as Thermage, which uses radio-frequency energy to firm and revitalize collagen.

If you've been bad, you could spend a lot of money to repair the damage. You may see further skin sagging and deeper dynamic wrinkles, especially if you've never had Botox. Your skin can look even duller with more brown spots. Your eyelids can sag, giving them a hooded appearance. And your skin will be drier. Some women have a genetic tendency toward excess skin draping their eyelids and may consider blepharoplasty (plastic surgery on the eyelids) as early as their late thirties.

Procedure	Frequency	Cost per treatment
Botox for the same 3 sites mentioned in previous section	Every 3–6 months	$700–$1,500
Fillers—Juvéderm, Perlane, Restylane, Cosmoderm, Cosmoplast, Radiesse, Sculptra—for lines around the mouth and "marionette" lines	1–2 syringes every 6–12 months	$1,000–$4,000
Maintenance IPL treatment	2–3 times per year	$400
Eye lift—blepharoplasty or Thermage	Once	$2,000–$4,000 for blepharoplasty; $1,500–$2,000 for Thermage
Thermage lift on face and/or neck	Every 2–3 years	$1,300–$6,000

Ages Sixty and Beyond

Menopause is past. If you have taken care of your skin, you're in pretty good shape. Age has left you with thinner skin and heavier wrinkling, but your inner beauty can still shine, and you are no longer challenged by fluctuating hormones. You may have bleeding under the skin that shows up as dark patches, especially on your hands, called purpura. At this time, some women are on blood thinners or daily aspirin to prevent heart disease, which exacerbates the problem. You could see sagging, skin tags (small, benign bits of skin that protrude from the underlying skin), and seborrheic keratosis, a common benign tumor that looks like a wart. Sagging can be addressed with Thermage or with a minimally invasive face-lift called an "S-lift," a procedure done under local anesthesia in which skin is excised in the shape of an S in front of the ears and the skin is tightened surgically. Growths can be treated with cryotherapy—frozen off with liquid nitrogen—every three to six months to keep things under control.

Maintain your daily vitamin and supplement regimen (omega-3s are all the more important at this stage, because they may increase mental functioning and memory), eat more wholegrain carbohydrates, continue with retinol treatments, and use topical antioxidants. If you've done most of the things we've already listed in years prior, the years to come will be a breeze. Protection from the sun plus maintenance equals lower skin-care costs and better results in later years. If you've avoided any additional sun damage, you can skip many of the photodamage treatments in this section. This will lower your costs. Your skin still needs more moisture, notwithstanding, and SPF protection is still a must.

Procedure	Frequency	Cost per treatment
Botox for the forehead, frown lines, and crow's-feet	Every 6 months (you need less frequent injections if you have had continued treatments over time)	$700–$1,500
Fillers as described previously (studies show using hylauronic acid fillers may stimulate collagen production)	1–2 syringes every 6–9 months	$600–$1,200
Radio-frequency treatment	Every 2–3 years	$1,300–$6,000
Maintenance IPL treatment	2–3 times per year	$400

If you live to eighty (we know you're going to be fabulous to one hundred), this all adds up to a tidy sum of money. Be thrifty

BEAUTY BUSTERS

Beauty myths debunked while you wait

Myth: Skin-care products are all hype.

Fact: This is a case of overhyped products and their critics tarring good ones with the same brush. Are there beauty products out there that are oversold? Yes. Does this mean that all beauty products are worthless? Certainly not. In the last twenty years, the science of skin care has grown tremendously; we now know more than ever about chemicals and natural compounds that deliver genuine benefits to the skin. We know that antioxidants are powerful agents for repairing damage to cells and their DNA inflicted by free radicals from the environment, stress, and pollution. We know that retinoids and alpha and beta hydroxy acids can reduce the appearance of wrinkles and photoaging and revitalize collagen. And we know that nutritional supplements, such as the polyphenols in green tea and the omega-3 fatty acids in salmon, help promote healthy skin. To bust this myth on your own, always know what's in the beauty products you buy. You read your food labels, don't you? If the ingredients of a skin-care product aren't listed, are unfamiliar, or make over-the-top promises, ask your dermatologist for an appraisal.

as well as beautiful: start taking better care of your skin today, and you'll be able to skip many of the procedures recommended for sun damage and wrinkles.

YOU BETTER SHOP AROUND

It's not good for your beauty to have your jaw sitting on the floor, so please pick it back up as we explain. Yes, that's a ton of money to spend on your beauty, and that's not even accounting for cosmetics, manicures, hairstyling, clothing, spas, and all the rest. We know that. We're not trying to produce an elitist book only for wealthy women. We want our solutions to be accessible to anyone. All the same, these are the hard facts on what premium beauty products and procedures cost today. This is a multibillion-dollar industry.

Let's first put the numbers in some perspective. Let's say you're forty years old and you're going to spend $500,000 by the time you're eighty on skin care, cosmetic treatments, hair care, makeup, and nails. That's $12,500 a year. But consider this: a British insurance company surveyed women in the United Kingdom and found that they will spend an average of about $54,000 on shoes in their lifetimes. That's for something that lasts maybe two years. Skin and hair are for life.

One thing you can count on: we're telling you about the good stuff. The products we recommend here are the products we recommend to our patients. There are times that prescription products are appropriate for your individual skin needs, and the products we mention often work in harmony with these. We also have the philosophy that less is more—and more is less. Any skin regimen requires a maximum of four individual products for any given day. If you are using more than that, more is actually less. When you apply layers of different products, less of the top layer is penetrating into the skin. Sometimes, layering can cancel out the efficacy of the products you are applying. So, always remember: less is more, including more savings on beauty products.

But what if you don't have thousands of dollars to spend each year on skin care? First of all, don't feel pressured to do all the things in the plan. You can do only what you can do, and the stress of going deep into credit card debt to pay for expensive procedures will damage your skin more than the procedures will

BEAUTY PEARLS

More than beauty, it is our own perception of beauty that constantly pushes us to strive for that "something" that defines us as beautiful beings, be it physically or spiritually. In the physical spectrum, being beautiful may be defined by perfect facial symmetry or by a gorgeous smile, but it is on the spiritual plane that beauty takes its true form. How to achieve it? Begin with a positive outlook in life and understand that there are more positives than negatives.

First and foremost, understand that beauty is in the eye of the beholder. Every woman in her uniqueness is beautiful. Nevertheless, a little help goes a long way—with emphasis on "little." Dramatic changes or extreme makeovers are not the answer. From this point of origin, there are three key factors to keep in mind:

*1. **Be informed.** New technologies, cosmetic breakthroughs, and innovative formulas are a part of our lives, and there is no reason why we should not be aware of them. Decisions are best made after ample research.*

*2. **Go through a mental checklist.** Or, in other words, do not leave the house without looking at yourself like your mother would. "Pillow hair" may be chic at seventeen, but not at thirty. Dedicate time to yourself; a little moisturizer, a dab of foundation, and a touch of mascara can do the trick in five minutes.*

*3. **Don't judge and don't fret.** There is nothing more beautiful than when you remember that you're not alone in this world. It is not only about you, but it is about who you are and what you can do for others. Beauty lies within, so being comfortable with who you are as a person radiates a special energy that translates into fewer frown lines, more luminosity, less weariness, and more smiles. How beautiful is that?*

—Ana Hughes-Freund, beauty editor,
Vogue Latinoamerica *and* Vogue Mexico

help it. Here are some other tips on getting the best skin care on your budget:

- **Shop around.** It's almost always possible to find discounts on some products, though you've got to be careful about low prices that compromise quality. Try looking on the Internet to locate the best deals available. You can also explore online options such as rebate clubs and e-coupons.
- **Take advantage of credit card rebates.** Some credit cards rebate a percentage of your annual purchases to you. Getting $1,000 back from your beauty purchases can take a little of the sting out.
- **Do the little things right.** Take care of your body, and you probably won't have to do as much. Exercise. Eat well. Get enough sleep. Drink water. Manage your stress level. Wear sunscreen. Take joy in life. Smile. This is all cheap or free and has a lot to do with how good you look and feel.
- **Talk to your dermatologist.** New products and options appear all the time. Ask your dermatologist if there are lower-cost alternatives to some of these products and treatments. Some dermatologists do in-office dispensing for their patients, and having this imprimatur can alleviate the guesswork.
- **Check out the drugstore.** Drugstore brands can help you save on skin care. Since the ingredients are what matters, always read the labels. Often, the only difference between a department-store brand and a drugstore brand is the packaging. In fact, some cosmetic companies have a drugstore brand and comparable department-store version. A 2007 *Consumer Reports* issue reviewed antiaging creams, and the one that came out on top was an Olay product, available over the counter at practically any drugstore.

• **Save and plan.** Save a little from every paycheck, and treat yourself to something for your beauty when you have the money. We love this option, because you get the microdermabrasion and the peace of mind that comes with knowing you're not going into debt. Try an automatic deduction from your checking account that puts aside a certain amount every two weeks for beauty. It adds up, and you don't have to think about it.

• **Give up a few things.** Check into what financial guru David Bach calls your "latte factor." Are there simple things you can give up or cut down on that will save you a lot of money over time? How much would you save if you quit smoking or cut your Starbucks trips in half? Twenty dollars a week adds up fast.

AN INNER BEAUTY PLAN

"But, Eva and Debra, that's only a program for the outside!" We hear you, and we're going to fix that. It's just as crucial to care for yourself on the inside, and the same basic requirement pertains to inner beauty as to outer: long-term commitment. Just as you need to apply SPF daily and exfoliate regularly, it's important to practice optimism and self-kindness over the long haul. Only when you attend to your mental and emotional health steadily over the years do you develop life-affirming habits and bring out your true inner beauty.

The Inner Beauty Plan comes with its own challenges. Unlike with skin care, it doesn't cost anything unless you choose to see a therapist at some point, but the results are also less obvious. With Botox, you can see a difference right away, whereas with affirmations or self-forgiveness, you might not notice any change in the way you see yourself, at least not immediately. It takes time for the difference to build. Give yourself a chance. You can make yourself into a more positive, loving, assertive, joyful woman by sheer will. Eventually, you start living a beautiful life, and that is really the ultimate goal.

Here's our Inner Beauty Plan:

- **Repeat affirmations.** Every day, at least once (preferably when you get up and go to sleep), repeat to yourself a set of verbal affirmations that remind you who you are and who you will become. Phrases such as "I am becoming healthier each day," "I am capable of handling whatever life brings my way," "I look forward to my day," and "I will see beauty in myself and others" are empowering.
- **Review positive moments.** Before you fall asleep, replay the positive moments from your day in your mind. This will store them so you can recall them when you wake up and start your day from a positive place.
- **Be in the moment.** Once each day, stop what you're doing and appreciate the moment. You don't have to be out hang gliding or watching Roger Federer play at the U.S. Open to do this; you could be in line at the market. What matters is that for a few seconds, you step out of the rushing stream of time and just be. Appreciate where you are and how extraordinary it is that you're alive at all. Look around you and realize that this particular moment will never come again. Find something to tuck away in your memory.
- **Catch one negative thought and change it.** Also daily, catch yourself having a negative thought about yourself, and reverse course. Instead of berating yourself or deciding that you can't do something, change your self-talk to something positive, empowering, and action oriented. You *can* do it. You *will* do it.

- **Challenge yourself to stop and find beauty.** Once a day, set what you're doing aside and spend a couple of minutes finding beauty in what's around you. Again, this doesn't mean you need to be cruising New England marveling at fall foliage. In fact, it's better if you challenge yourself to find beauty in unexpected places, maybe a downtown construction scene. Doing so sharpens your sense of beauty and your ability to locate it in any situation. It also makes the world brighter and friendlier.
- **Find one thing about you that's beautiful.** Once a week, remind yourself of one thing about you that's beautiful. It could be something obvious, such as your eyes, or something unseen, perhaps your sense of humor. Don't take it for granted. Tell yourself out loud: "Hey, lady, you have great cheekbones." Try to find something beautiful about yourself each week that's different from the week before. Before long, you'll start seeing whole new aspects of you as beautiful.
- **Commit random kindnesses.** Once a week, do something thoughtful for someone you don't know, with no provocation or expectation of reward. Pay for the movie tickets of the couple in front of you in line. Trim the garden of the elderly lady in your neighborhood who's too frail to do it herself. Find something beautiful in a stranger, and tell her you see it. The best way to feel wonderful about yourself, and life in general, is to bring light into the lives of others. Try it. It's addictive in the best possible way.
- **Take a risk.** Once a month, try something new that's outside your comfort zone. Make it something at which you have a decent chance of succeeding, because taking a risk and coming through with flying colors is fantastic for your confidence and self-esteem. This could be speaking in public, or it could be making plans with someone you've admired for a while. The possibilities are there for the taking.

• **Express your gratitude.** At the end of each day, remind yourself of all the things that happened during the day for which you should be grateful. Maybe you visited your mother, completed a project at work, or got a clean bill of health after a physical. Be thankful. Taking life's good fortune for granted is a path to cynicism. Life can change on a dime, so appreciate everything and everyone you have.

The path to inner beauty begins with these steps just as surely as outer beauty resides in regular skin care and guarding your health. Living a beautiful life is a plan—and firm dedication and commitment—away.

Beauty Bullets

ᐧᐧᐧ Society considers older women to be beautiful.

ᐧᐧᐧ You need a long-term commitment for any plan to work.

ᐧᐧᐧ The proper use of sunscreen is essential to maintain outer beauty as well as health.

ᐧᐧᐧ Good skin care is expensive, but there are ways to save.

ᐧᐧᐧ A lifetime program for inner beauty is also vital.

ᐧᐧᐧ For both inner and outer beauty, lifelong discipline is necessary to see results.

BEAUTY AND THE BRAIN Rx

Be a Quitter

Dr. Eva: *Please, if you smoke, quit. There are few worse things a woman can do for her health and beauty than smoke cigarettes. According to the American Lung Association, smoking-related disease takes 430,700 American lives each year and is by far the major cause of lung cancer, which is the leading cancer killer of women in the United States. There is nothing good about this habit. If you do nothing else to enhance your beauty, quit smoking. Some tips from the American Lung Association:*

- *Join a stop-smoking program such as Freedom From Smoking.*
- *Check into self-help options such as guidebooks, videotapes, and audiotapes. Such materials are available from the ALA.*
- *Pick a time to quit when you're not under stress or in a lot of social situations.*
- *Be aware that smokers have different experiences as their bodies go through nicotine withdrawal. Some get sleepy. Others eat. Others get headaches.*
- *Get some exercise daily. This helps reduce the stress of quitting and helps prevent weight gain, common with quitting.*
- *Get plenty of sleep, eat a balanced diet, and hydrate.*
- *Ask family and friends to help. Set up Beauty Buddies you can call when you're tempted to light up.*
- *Talk with your doctor about prescription medications that help smokers resist nicotine cravings and quit more successfully.*
- *Consider hypnosis or acupuncture—anything that will help you, especially the first few weeks.*

Dr. Debra: *Not only does smoking cause lung cancer, but also, other than sun exposure, it's the worst thing you can do to your skin. Ever notice women with lines that radiate from the lips? Lipstick tends to bleed into these lines, making them even more obvious. They are caused by smoking. Of all the cosmetic issues women have, this is the most difficult one to treat. Smoking also contributes to a spotty, dull complexion. Furthermore, if you have any thoughts about getting plastic surgery, most plastic surgeons will insist you stop smoking, because the risk of complications—including poor healing and anesthesia related death—goes up exponentially. And yellow teeth and smoker's breath don't exactly enhance your outer beauty.*

9

Beauty 911: Being Your Best During Times of Transition

There is in every true woman's heart a spark of
heavenly fire, which lies dormant in the broad daylight
of prosperity, but which kindles up and beams and
blazes in the dark hour of adversity.

—Washington Irving

IN THIS CORNER, wearing the red silk trunks, we have Ancient Saying Number One: "Adversity builds character." In the other corner, wearing the blue trunks with the gold trim, we have Ancient Saying Number Two: "Adversity doesn't build character; it reveals it." We're going to let these two duke it out while we propose a third, beauty-centric alternative: Adversity tests beauty.

It's much easier to be beautiful when things are peachy. When everybody's healthy, and money is in the bank, and the marriage is solid, and the kids are doing well in school or are grown and on their own, life seems more joyful and satisfying. With no crisis to manage, you have more time to invest in your inner and outer beauty: exercising, volunteering, meditating, doing the things that make your life beautiful. Then, when crisis crashes through, as it does for all of us, your appearance and the entire Beauty-Brain Loop can take a pummeling. When a health problem befalls you or someone in your sphere, or when difficulties with money or a relationship emerge, the stress of the experience and the demands of managing it can mean beauty is abandoned like an old car by the side of the road.

It doesn't have to be that way. It is possible to protect your inner and outer beauty even during life's most challenging stages. Just have a Beauty 911 plan, and when the going gets tough, don't hesitate to put it into action.

TIMES OF TRANSITION

What we're really talking about here are life's inevitable transition periods, when change is wrenching and abrupt and leaves you gasping. Sure, sometimes crisis comes out of nowhere, such as with accidents or a natural disaster, but those events are comparatively rare. In the majority of cases, the most stressful periods in any woman's life will be transition periods:

- Death of a loved one
- Placing an aging parent in a care facility
- Divorce
- Infidelity or other marital problems
- Retirement
- Menopause
- Health troubles—yours or a loved one's
- Job loss or financial crisis
- Children leaving home
- Moving

BEAUTY BUDDIES

Shannon Griefer, forty-seven, and Meryl Brown, forty-five

Shannon is a former couch potato who discovered distance running when she was in her thirties and has now become an elite ultramarathoner—the first woman to "double" the murderous Badwater 135 race through Death Valley, running a total of 292 miles in a single race. Now she's inspired her friend of twenty-five years, Meryl, to become a mega-distance runner, too.

"Meryl is the kind of woman that other women hate, because she can eat a bag of Cheetos and not gain an ounce," Shannon says. "I got Meryl into running. She is really fast, and she eventually qualified for the Boston Marathon, ran her first 50K, and later ran her first 50-mile race. Now she's getting her certification as a personal trainer, coaching other people and helping them learn to run. I think she's inspiring."

"Shannon has changed my life," Meryl says. "My life would never be the same without her. Everywhere I run, they know Shannon. Everybody I know is in awe of her." Shannon adds, "Now that we're both into being healthy and fit, we're hoping to inspire others. People usually do things for themselves, but we want to do this for others and help them run."

As you might guess, running is Shannon and Meryl's Beauty Buddy activity. Rather than run on the streets, they like to go deep into the backcountry and run for miles, letting the beauty and solitude work its magic on them. "We run in the mountains and talk about our lives and how beautiful the world is," says Shannon. "It's a really beautiful place. We go out to the mountains, drop supplies of water that we can drink as we return on the trail, and hope the mountain lions don't follow us. We talk about our lives and what we were doing about twenty-five years ago and how much healthier our lives are now."

Meryl ties it all together: "You don't have a friend for twenty-five years unless you're really lucky. Our running is the big tie in our friendship. Everything is about our runs and our kids and what we're going to do next."

Transitions upset our equilibrium, and that sense is compounded by grief and worry that may linger for weeks or months. A frequent and understandable consequence is that we let ourselves go. Who has time to worry about such trifles as hair and nails when the world is spinning out of control? To top it off, harsh transitions can provoke a host of potentially debilitating physical reactions:

- Fatigue, shakes, dizziness, and heart palpitations
- Difficulty breathing and chest pains
- Nausea, diarrhea, and vomiting
- Muscular tension, headaches, and neck and back pain
- Increased or decreased sexual desire and activity
- Anxiety or panic attacks
- Insomnia or the desire to sleep excessively

Between the racket in the mind and the coiled, oppressive tension in the body, it can be a chore to muster an ounce of concern about how you look during a harsh life transition. While we both sympathize, we'd argue that a crisis is exactly when you should devote extra attention to protecting your beauty inside and out.

STOP THE CAROUSEL—I WANT TO GET OFF!

A woman who had been a regular patient for Botox and dermal fillers came to see Debra for more of the same. Asked how she was doing, she said that things weren't so good: she had been diagnosed with colon cancer and was about to have surgery. Why the cosmetic procedures, a seemingly insignificant matter compared with cancer? "I want to look my best going into this fight," she said. Like a warrior preparing for battle, she was putting on her armor. In a situation in which she lacked control, this was one part she could control.

This is the most important reason to have a Beauty 911 plan: to recapture a sense of control in your life at a time when structures seem to be spiraling downward on their own accord. A sense of control is vital to one's well-being. When something goes wrong in your life and the earth seems to be spinning like a carousel with you hanging on for dear life, how you look and feel may be the only aspect you *can* control. We soothe ourselves with the idea that life is somehow predictable and that people get what they deserve, but that's largely illusory. Stuff happens. Bad things happen to good people.

When they do, one of the life preservers within your reach is good self-care—dressing well, knowing that your skin and hair look good, managing the effects of stress, and having enough self-esteem to say, "I will get through this."

YOUR BEAUTY 911 PLAN

When the marriage of Brad Pitt and Jennifer Aniston broke up in early 2005, Aniston was understandably devastated. Nobody would have faulted her if she had chosen to hide in her home and spend Oscar night in her sweats eating Oreos. Instead, she dressed to the nines in black with pearls, walked the red carpet, and presented the award for Best Costume Design. Rather than cower and grieve, she chose to get gorgeous and show the world that she was still a beautiful, desirable young woman.

That's breaking out your Beauty 911 plan and working it. The Beauty 911 plan is a strategy for staying as beautiful as pos-

BEAUTY PEARLS

We become beautiful when we're in touch with who we really are and when we, as women, are in control of our financial lives. In my research among women and financially successful Americans—from Oprah to the newly minted millionaire around the corner—I've found a few key truths. The first is that the more we give, the more we get. Giving goes beyond the physical or intellectual act of contributing of our time or mind; it gets to something deeper, more emotional. When we give, we feel valued as humans and that, in turn, translates into both inner and outer beauty. That's why one of the keys in my book, The Millionaire Zone, *is Getting by Giving. We can give in myriad ways, from mentoring and offering advice to making introductions and providing financial or emotional support to some person or cause.*

I'm also a big believer—especially for women—that when we have control over our financial lives, we radiate confidence and beauty. Time after time I see women who have to stay in relationships because they need to, not because they want to. I see them stay in jobs that hold them back rather than propel them forward. I see them giving up on their dreams rather than pursuing them. Women will ultimately live happier lives if they have the freedom and ability to make the choices they want. And that requires having a partner who respects you as an economic equal. It also means that women have to be active participants and invest for their futures. In the end, they'll have less stress, more fulfilling relationships, and a stronger sense of self. Now that's beautiful!

—Jennifer Openshaw, author, The Millionaire Zone; *president, WeSeeds.com; national financial commentator for Fox, AOL, and ABC Radio*

sible even when life turns you upside down. It's a collection of mental and emotional advice, reminders, and beauty tips to help you take care of your skin, hair, and overall health when things are a little crazy and you just want to scream.

As Jennifer Aniston discovered, not surrendering to the anger, despair, or pain not only makes you feel more in control but gives you perspective to boot. When you realize that in spite of the bad news or the terrible circumstances, you can still look good and feel strong, you see that in the end, this too shall pass. No crisis lasts forever. There is healing at the end of the road. You will get through this and still be you.

The power of the Beauty 911 plan is that when you're at your worst and you can barely think straight, it does your thinking for you. You're prepared to take on whatever comes along, because the plan guides you in caring for your skin, your self-esteem, and your emotional health. You most likely have insurance to cover you in case of a fire, a health problem, a car accident, or an injury on the job. Think of this as insurance for your inner and outer beauty. It isn't just Boy Scouts who are prepared. Girl Scouts should be, too.

Danger or Opportunity?

In a speech in 1959, John F. Kennedy said, "When written in Chinese the word *crisis* is composed of two characters. One represents danger and the other represents opportunity." That's a perfect summation of the choice you have when you're waylaid by the overpowering stress of a crisis situation. As we've discussed, true self-esteem comes not from "I'm a special person" statements but from actual accomplishments in which you dis-

BEAUTY STORY: "ALLISON"

Allison, forty-eight, came to see Debra about six months after the sudden death of her husband. She complained that she felt the way she looked: "twenty years older than I am." As they spoke about Botox, fillers, and skin care, Debra noted how often Allison mentioned her late husband and became emotional. Concluding that Allison's self-critical attitude was part of her mourning process, she made the gentle suggestion that Allison talk to a therapist.

In sessions with a psychologist, Allison revealed that she had been blaming herself for her husband's death because she hadn't urged him to take care of his health. Letting beauty slide and criticizing herself for looking old was a way of punishing herself. Her therapist suggested some cognitive exercises as well as other activities—such as joining a grief support group—to bring her out of this nonproductive cycle of guilt. Over the following year, she returned to a healthy beauty process and appeared to be handling her grief in a more constructive fashion.

Eva: People who have never experienced real grief, including those in the midst of it for the first time, usually fail to understand how long the process takes and what it's like—for the grieving party as well as others. There aren't any rules. You don't "get over" the loss of a loved one; you learn to live with the loss. What Allison needed more than anything was a therapist to listen to her and help her become aware of her thought processes. In therapy, she was able to recognize that her guilt was misplaced and to feel better about herself.

Debra: She came back to see me about nine months after that first appointment, and the difference was astounding. She had been taking care of her skin, exercising, and getting some rest, and it showed in every aspect of her appearance. I asked her how she was, and she replied simply, "Healing."

covered your strengths. When crisis or trauma descends, your self-esteem is put to the test. Do you have the reserves of strength to prevail? Can you draw on lessons from past crises to confront this latest one?

The potent and often unrelenting stress of a health, marital, or financial storm can do a number on your self-esteem. You may doubt your ability to cope. You might dwell on the negative, seeing doom where it does not exist and rendering yourself incapable of arriving at a solution. You could blame yourself for a situation that is not your fault. The sheer weight of a traumatic event can confound your sense of reality and perspective, leaving you convinced that there is only darkness ahead, or leaving you feeling isolated and hopeless. This sequence can foster depression, a much more serious condition.

Having a Beauty 911 plan in place is a blessing in a situation like this. You know that something is not out of control. You do have the power to cope and to keep yourself looking good and feeling healthy. If you're thinking, "Come on, what does it matter if my hair is properly styled if my father has just been diagnosed with Alzheimer's?" Even if it doesn't matter to you, it matters to other people. In a crisis, people are looking for someone to take the lead, ask the tough questions, and lend comfort. As women, we're nurturers, and offering comfort often falls to us. How will you convey confidence and leadership to others who need it if you look disheveled and exhausted? By looking good and standing tall, you can give others a firmer sense of order in a disorderly time—and it can help make you *feel* that you deserve to be in control.

So, to address JFK's issue of danger versus opportunity, we say: look out for both. When crisis erupts, if your self-esteem is already weak, you're going to have a rough time, but if it's strong, you can take action to reveal the opportunity in the danger—to discover your true strength and resiliency. That's really a smart woman's way of making the best of a bad situation.

INNER BEAUTY AND CALAMITY

The emotions connected to a traumatic event—even if it's something expected, such as the finalization of a divorce or moving from your home of thirty years—can stimulate a stress response that is devastating. Just imagine what it must be like to survive something sudden and catastrophic, such as Hurricane Katrina! In a crisis situation of any magnitude, your mind can become your worst enemy.

Certain emotions are normal and expected in response to a crisis, and you may rapidly shift between a wide range of reactions:

* **Shock and disbelief:** This often emerges first. The event seems to be unreal, like a film or a dream. You may keep thinking you will wake up and it will be over.
* **Numbness:** Your emotions seem muffled or turned off. Nothing brings you pleasure, and life may seem meaningless.
* **Fear:** You may worry excessively about death, injury, or harm to yourself or loved ones. You may become fearful of being left alone or leaving others, of breaking down, or of experiencing a recurrence of the event.
* **Helplessness:** You may feel powerless to cope with the situation. Sadness can become consuming, and crying is common.
* **Longing:** You yearn for things that are gone or will never be.
* **Guilt:** You chastise yourself for having survived, for not having done enough to help others, or for not being better to others.

• **Anger:** You rail against God, fate, injustice, the senselessness of what happened, someone who acted wrongly, indignities, red tape, or lack of understanding by others.

Imagine having many of these conflicting emotions at the same time, all the time, for days or weeks without a break. Many people wrap themselves in family or support groups to help them survive the nonstop stress. That's a good idea. Healthy coping mechanisms should be part of every woman's beauty arsenal. Others may turn to alcohol or drugs to dull their emotions. That course is sure to make things worse instead of better.

So Much More than Sad

We all feel angry, sad, anxious, or self-defeating sometimes. While those feelings are normal, failing to confront a crisis in a constructive way can leave you feeling helpless, hopeless, or continually fearful and panicked. This is why having cognitive control is germane to inner beauty. Since what you think controls how you feel, telling yourself, "I don't think I can get through this" can become a self-fulfilling prophecy for personal powerlessness. Thoughts become habits, with their own neural pathways in the brain. When you allow a life trauma to become a source of endless stress and fear, it's a short drop off a cliff into depression and anxiety disorders.

Depression

Depression can be the result of life events such as the death of a loved one or divorce. Scientists don't fully understand why overwhelming stress leads to depression in some people while others

BEAUTY BOOSTERS

Practical things you can do now to be more beautiful

Cultivate a passion, something you could do all night without feeling tired, something you would do for the rest of your life even if you were never paid a dime for it. Many people have buried their passions in favor of practical considerations, but that's foolish. We need passion to bring joy and meaning to living. Ask yourself, what do you love to do? What activity or goal brings energy and purpose to your day? It could be volunteering or mentoring, or something domestic such as cooking or landscaping your yard. It doesn't matter, as long as it's something that resonates deep inside you. Find out what your passion is, and devote some of your time and energy to it. The joy and gratitude you derive from spending some of your time living passionately will spill over into the rest of your life, enhancing your inner beauty and spreading positive energy throughout the loop.

are able to bounce back after a certain time. Clinical depression is not "the blues." It is a serious illness that stems from complex chemical imbalances in the brain and affects the lives of about twelve million U.S. women each year, according to the National Institute of Mental Health. One in four American women will experience depression at some time.

Symptoms include sadness, irritability, decreased concentration, change in appetite, loss of interest in previously enjoyed activities, insomnia or oversleeping, and sometimes even thoughts of suicide.

Often, untreated depression will go away with time, but in other cases, treatment is necessary. Nobody should self-diagnose a negative mood and elect to forgo treatment of this potentially dangerous disease. Studies have shown psychotherapy to be effective for lifting depression. Antidepressant medications likewise can be effective and can be used in conjunction with therapy to help the patient gain greater control over moods.

Social support has also been shown to be of value in alleviating the symptoms of depression, while studies in England suggest that couples' counseling is as of much benefit as medication for treating depression. In the end, there are many options for dealing with depression, but there are no "off-the-rack" solutions. Only a mental health professional can help people determine if they are suffering from depression and how best to treat the condition.

Anxiety

Anxiety disorders also affect millions of American women and, as with depression, do so at a greater rate than for men. The reasons for the disparity are still poorly understood, but most likely, hormones play a role in our greater susceptibility.

Anxiety disorders are a common affliction in modern cultures where women have many roles and little support. Many women become anxious, worry excessively, and have difficulty sleeping. These problems can worsen as we grow older and life becomes more complicated. Perimenopause, the interval before true menopause when physical changes begin, is fertile ground for anxiety, depression, personality changes, and sleep disturbances.

The most common anxiety disorders are the following:

• **Generalized anxiety disorder:** You worry about things all the time, even when there's no justification for it. Crisis can create the impression that such fears are justified.

- **Panic disorder:** This frightening disorder brings on sudden, baseless feelings of terror and imminent doom. You may experience a racing heart, chills, chest pain, and the feeling that something terrible is about to happen. Again, crisis can reinforce this belief and make symptoms worse.

- **Social anxiety disorder:** This disorder makes it difficult to be around other people in even the most benign social situations. You might feel that everyone is watching and judging you, which can lead to sweating, trembling, and nausea and even to avoidance of social situations.

Anxiety has been shown to respond to a variety of treatments, including yoga, meditation, psychotherapy, medication, and change of environment. The hitch is that before anxiety can be treated, it must be identified, and many women don't even know that the persistent worry or social phobia from which they suffer is a diagnosable and treatable illness. Anxiety can cripple your life under the weight of fear, but self-awareness can reduce your risk of developing it.

A PINK BELT IN KINDNESS

Time does not heal all wounds. That's a myth, but when you're in the throes of grief or regret after a rough transition, inaction isn't going to make you feel much better, either. We've both treated women right after divorce or discovering infidelity or other relationship problems, and their feelings of betrayal and loss do not just abate over weeks and months. Time helps, but positive, life-affirming measures help more.

"A big part of what I do is help women to find ways to cope with something that is unfamiliar to them," says Christina Pozo-

Kaderman, Ph.D., codirector of Psychosocial Services at Mount Sinai Comprehensive Cancer Center, in Miami. She counsels cancer patients in both behavioral and emotional recovery methods, which makes her an expert on keeping a sense of beauty during rough times. "If they're young," she notes, "they've never had something so big to cope with before. I find ways to use the coping methods they already have."

What does Pozo-Kaderman recommend as most healing for her patients? "Find ways to express your emotions. Find interests and hobbies and things you feel a passion for. Try to be present in the moment, practicing mindfulness. Slow down. Try to take things in and be present. Really taste what you're eating, really walk outside and breathe in and see what things smell like. Don't take things for granted."

BEAUTY BUSTERS

Beauty myths debunked while you wait

Myth: Crying is unhealthy.
Fact: There are healthy and unhealthy expressions of grief. Whereas avoidance is an unhealthy expression, there is nothing wrong with a good cry. Crying acts as a pressure release valve for the emotions, allowing us to let off some of what we are feeling, be it anger, fear, or sadness. So, when something sad happens, go ahead and let yourself have a "good" cry. Do it alone or with someone by your side. However, crying that doesn't stop or that comes on out of the blue may indicate depression. That's a sign for a woman that she needs extra help in coping with the stress or loss and should speak with a mental health professional.

Cancer is a wake-up call for women, she says, one that other women should heed. "They realize how much they are loved, which they didn't realize before. They realize they had strength they never knew they had." She adds, " I have had women, once they recovered, leave relationships that didn't work for them. They know they can deal with anything that life brings them."

In a traumatic situation, the first commandment is to be kind to yourself. Don't blame or torture yourself with guilt, and don't play the "what-if" game. What's done is done. Be forgiving, and remind yourself that you're doing the best you can. Beyond that, think of positive approaches you can take to heal and move beyond the situation at hand, and then take action. Sometimes, just doing what's practically necessary makes you feel as if you've emerged from some sort of cocoon of grief.

We know a woman who, while her husband lay in an intensive care unit near death, pulled herself out of her fear long enough to contact the company that held her 401(k) and learn about the taxes and penalties involved in withdrawing the money. She knew that if her husband died, the grief and necessity to care for their children would leave her unable to work for some time. So, she prepared. Fortunately, her husband recovered, but we commend her for taking action. She assumed control during rough waters. Even if a crisis doesn't end in death, divorce, or bankruptcy, it's still vital to act, lest you spend years worrying, "What if it happens again?" When you act and prepare, worry fades.

This may seem like contradictory advice, but it's really not: be patient. OK, which is it: act now, or wait around? Both, actually. Definitely do constructive things to manage through crisis, but don't expect to feel all better right away. This is when friends with the best intentions can do more harm than good. Grief makes others uncomfortable; they want you to "just get over it" for their sakes as much as for your own. Remember those mirror neurons? It's painful to watch someone else suffering, and it's natural to want them to feel better as quickly as possible. It's also a fact, however, that when you bury your grief or fear beneath layers of denial, you can't heal. Grief will rise up and catch you, believe us. Take your time. It can be years before you get past the powerful emotions stirred up by a distressing experience.

Your inner beauty will come through hard times far more intact if you give yourself time and a lot of love. Protecting your inner beauty during periods of stress is not easy, but it will pay off in the long run as you learn to face up to life's challenges more adeptly. True self-confidence comes from knowing we can dispatch all that life throws at us.

DON'T DROWN YOUR SORROWS

You're not Karen Allen in *Raiders of the Lost Ark*, drinking a huge Tibetan under the table and then getting up as if she'd been shooting plain water (which she probably was). When you're in the middle of a crisis, you are extremely vulnerable, because a part of you is rejecting your new reality and looking for a way out. In these circumstances, it is not difficult to wind up abusing drugs or, more commonly, alcohol. For your own sake, don't. Don't drink when you're struggling through a wrenching transition.

First of all, alcohol exacerbates the body's reaction to stress, which can worsen skin and general health problems. Second, drinking or taking drugs will impair your ability to make judgments in a difficult situation. Third, alcohol disrupts sleep, leaving you less well equipped to cope with challenges the next day. It also alters the chemistry in the brain, making you more susceptible to anxiety or depressive disorders. If you regularly use controlled substances, you will become addicted. And finally, using alcohol or any drug to blunt your crisis experience and run away from its implications denies you the ability to develop new coping skills, meaning you are more likely to experience problems in the next crisis. So, when a friend suggests that she come by with a bottle of cabernet and a DVD, tell her to come over but bring mineral water instead.

When to Get Help

Another carved-in-stone commandment of Beauty 911 is to lean on others. You're not a superhero. You don't have to go it alone, and you shouldn't. Remember, we're the social sex. We are far better than men at going to doctors, and we live longer. Think that's just a coincidence? Get support from friends, clergy, family, or coworkers. Talking with others is a wonderful way to get a fresh perspective. Ask a therapist: talking helps. It dislodges those unfounded fears and concerns from inside your skull and articulates them, shrinking them down to size. When you're under attack by life, form a circle and hold hands.

Sometimes, of course, informal help by well-meaning people isn't enough. Perhaps you have emotions you can't control or start to experience strange behavior such as obsessiveness or anxiety. That's when you might want to consider seeing a mental health professional. Therapy has been proved to work by helping new neurons fire and new pathways form in the brain. Different chemicals are then secreted by the brain, making you feel better and think more clearly. New ways of thinking can refurbish the brain and help you interact with your environment in new, healthier ways.

Let's get one thing straight: seeing a therapist does not mean you are mentally ill. It does not mean something is wrong with you. In fact, it means something is right. You are self-aware and wise enough to know you can't solve all your problems on your own. You are smart enough to ask for assistance. Therapy creates a safe, totally confidential space where you can receive objective, noncritical advice about the thoughts, feelings, and behaviors that are bothering you. It's an opportunity to talk to someone who won't tell you just what you want to hear, but who will give you space and encouragement to grow.

We would love to get rid of the stigma attached to seeing a mental health professional. We'd like to see it become as simple and routine as getting a mammogram: "Just place your head against this plate, Ms. Jones." Alas, it's never going to be that mechanical, but it doesn't have to be complicated, either. Here's a who's who of mental health:

- A psychiatrist is an M.D. who went to medical school and can do therapy and prescribe medication.
- A psychologist is a Ph.D. who studied the mind and can do therapy and testing to make the correct diagnosis.
- An L.C.S.W. or L.M.F.T. is a licensed clinical social worker or licensed marriage and family therapist. Both are professionals with a master's degree, trained in providing psychotherapy.

Choose a mental health professional the same way you would select any other service provider of value and importance: by referral. Talk with friends or family who have seen a therapist. Get a referral from your primary care physician, ob-gyn, or dermatologist. Ask lots of questions of prospective providers. Check out credentials on the Internet. Also, find out if your insurance covers mental health care (most do these days). Most of all, once you're in the room with your therapist, don't expect an instant fix. Therapy takes time, and you'll be doing the work. Your therapist is there to help you become more aware of your issues and your solutions. A good mental health professional can help you regain a sense of perspective during and after periods of crisis. The service provided translates to help in recovering and preserving your inner beauty.

Strong Is Beautiful

Some of the most beautiful women we've ever seen are women who have survived trauma, such as breast cancer or childhood abuse. When we see them in our offices or our lives, we're always intrigued by their beauty and strength. These are women who have seen the darkest times a person can see and have come out the other side into the light. There's a knowing in them that says, "I have the strength to get through anything." That's stunning.

Life is a challenge, but it's also an adventure. If there's not something difficult in your life right now, it's coming. Count on it. The secret to beauty is living a beautiful life, inside and out, with yourself and your community and the world around you. Women are sometimes raised to believe in the fairy tale of marrying a rich prince and living happily ever after, but buying into those fantasies only leaves you flailing when you encounter bumps in the road. You're among girlfriends, so let's be honest: the only one responsible for looking after you is *you*. Living a beautiful life demands finding the strength to be resilient and bounce back when life knocks you down. What separates truly beautiful women from the rest is that they bounce back, keep going, and re-embrace life with passion. That's strength, and that's beautiful.

Strength is taking full responsibility for your life and your beauty, making every part of your life the best it can be. The parts you can change, you change. The parts that are beyond your control, you accept. At the same time, you prepare yourself so that when the roller coaster drops, you're still on board when it rises back to the top. As women, we have more possibilities to create our lives than at any time in history. For example, more women serve on the boards of directors of Fortune 500 companies than ever before. There are more ways than ever for women to create amazing lives and maintain healthy bodies and minds. Yes, there are challenges in some parts of the world that would rather see women become invisible again, but it's not going to happen. We're not going anywhere. It's an exciting time. When life rains down on you, try to see the beauty in it, and remember that things will get better.

Your Inner Beauty 911 toolkit:

- **Learn to set limits.** Say no. Women are caretakers, but sometimes we have to draw the line. When times are hard, your limits are closer. Know when to stop being the one who is always taking care of others. Don't expect yourself to do everything during times of high stress. Pace yourself, and do what you can, and don't expect anything more.
- **Let yourself be vulnerable.** It's OK to cry and be afraid. Let other people take care of you.
- **Have people around.** Don't sit in an empty house worrying or grieving. Have friends or family over. Let them help with the

laundry, make dinner, or watch the kids. Let them hug you and listen to you. Love is therapy.

- **Don't assume trouble will pass you by.** It won't. Death strikes every family, and half of marriages end in divorce court. Something's going to happen sooner or later. Don't fret about the possibility, but be prepared.

- **Rest.** Get your sleep. When you're sleep deprived, you make poorer judgment calls, and your emotions are less under control.

- **Stay as positive as possible.** Positive emotions encourage action and reduce stress, helping you stay functioning as things play out.

- **Think through choices carefully.** Emotions sometimes lead us to make poor decisions in the heat of the moment. Step back and take your time with any important choice: care facilities, legal agreements, and so on.

- **Remember happy times.** Recalling good times spent with a person who's died can brighten your mood and keep that person alive in your heart. Reliving times that were happier will remind you that "this too shall pass" and that you will have happy times again.

- **Don't go to bed and think in circles.** Talk to someone. If you have fears or unresolved issues, speak to a support person about the conflict. Lying awake solves nothing and only makes you exhausted.

- **Be spiritual.** Whether you speak to God or meditate on Oneness, get in touch with your spiritual side. You'll derive comfort and strength from it.

- **Be kind to others.** Reach out to someone and remind yourself who you are: a beautiful woman who will come through your transition a stronger person.

- **Read.** Bookstores are filled with advice on how to steer through all types of choppy waters. Learning from others can help you along your journey.
- **Work the loop.** Remember that inner beauty relates to all other areas of the loop. Don't neglect your outer beauty or health, and allow your environment to nurture you to its fullest potential.

OUTER BEAUTY AND TRANSITION

In a provocative study, women suffering from depression experienced a reduction in their symptoms after receiving Botox to remove frown lines. It's not that we are advocating Botox for depression, but often when people look better, they really do feel better about themselves. Perhaps the environment responded more favorably to these women when they looked brighter and no longer came across as sad or angry. Perhaps a complex feedback system operates between the facial muscles and the brain. All the reasons aren't fully understood, but the link is clear: inner beauty and outer beauty are close cousins. Taking care of both is more effective than just taking care of one or the other, especially in times of crisis. Knowing that you look good in spite of everything that's falling apart will give you a feeling of confidence. You'll think, "Wow, I look pretty good. I can handle this problem."

Take proactive steps to protect your beauty when times are tough. Your stress response kicks in when adversity arrives, flooding your body with adrenaline and cortisol. These floods can agitate underlying skin conditions, such as rosacea, psoriasis, acne, or eczema. Follow these steps to safeguard your appearance when you're under stress:

- Take a day off from the demands of the situation if you can. Do nothing.
- Exercise. Working out increases your metabolism and keeps good hormones such as endorphins flowing, balancing your mood. It also gives you a time to try to clear your mind of worries.
- Avoid pro-inflammatory foods that increase cortisol levels— alcohol, caffeine, sugars, and simple starches.
- Include fish oils in your diet either by eating fish such as salmon and mackerel or by taking supplements. They have been shown to be mood stabilizers and are also good for your skin.
- Pamper yourself with a facial, spa treatment, or massage.
- Take a steamy shower. This doubles your pleasure, dilating blood vessels so your skin glows and relaxing you at the same time.
- Have your hair and nails done. The hands-on therapy does wonders for relaxation and can give you a quick dose of self-esteem.
- Dress up. During a crisis, dress *better* than you normally would. Exhibiting some flair makes you feel elegant and in charge and compels others to respond to you in the same way.

By taking these steps to manage stress and keep yourself healthy, you increase your odds of emerging from your tribulations looking and feeling like the strong, beautiful woman you are.

Now you have your Beauty 911 plan for inner and outer beauty. Keep it safe and handy in case things go south. Transitions are a part of life, but with preparation, they will only increase your self-esteem and give you an opportunity to show others what true beauty really is—inside and out.

Beauty Bullets

Ᏸ Adversity tests beauty.

Ᏸ Transition and difficult times are inevitable.

Ᏸ Crisis produces predictable mental and physical effects.

Ᏸ Depression or anxiety may need the attention of a professional who is trained to administer to these conditions.

Ᏸ Don't smoke.

Ᏸ Protect your outer beauty by following a healthy routine and thereby enhance your sense of control during difficult times.

 ## BEAUTY AND THE BRAIN Rx

Stress

Dr. Eva: In times of crisis, women may engage in "cognitive distortions," which are maladaptive patterns of thinking that affect how you interpret events in your world. For example, a woman may think that bad things keep happening to her because of some misdeed she committed. Or she may feel she deserves bad things to happen to her, or she anticipates bad things happening even when everything is fine. Your cognitive distortions can rob you of your optimism and keep you from making the changes you need to make.

Under stress, we tend to think less clearly because the primary centers of our brains are activated, overriding our reason. Some common examples of cognitive distortions include:

(continued)

- ***All-or-nothing thinking:*** *"My life is horrible and it will never get any better."*

- ***Personalization:*** *"I didn't get the job because I was too pushy," when in fact you didn't get the job because the boss gave it to his cousin.*

For more examples and a workbook to help you identify your cognitive distortions, read Feeling Good: The New Mood Therapy *by psychiatrist Dr. David D. Burns. It's a terrific guide to this kind of thinking and how to manage it.*

Distortions are poison for self-esteem because they turn the events, conflicts, and minor problems of everyday living into monsters. Cognitive behavioral therapy (CBT) has been shown to improve the clarity of your thinking and lift your mood. Learning to identify the mistakes you are making and replacing negative thoughts with constructive thoughts is at the heart of CBT.

Dr. Debra: *When the brain perceives stress, a cascade of hormonal responses ensues. First, the hypothalamus signals the pituitary gland, which then tells the adrenal glands to produce androgens and cortisol, powerful stress hormones. These hormones help thicken the lining of hair follicles, causing blackheads or whiteheads. The sebaceous glands also produce more oil, aggravating outbreaks. But acne is the tip of the iceberg. Chronic stress can bring on hives, eczema, psoriasis, rosacea, warts, cold sores, and blisters. The stress response also robs the skin of oxygen, which can make it look dull and lifeless.*

Manage stress to prevent skin problems. Exercise, meditation, deep breathing, and simply looking at beauty are optimal ways to prevent your body's response to stress from damaging your skin. Get enough sleep, and eat a diet rich in antioxidants, which help cleanse stress-produced free radicals from your body.

10

Secrets to Lending Nature a Hand

I was going to have cosmetic surgery until I noticed
that the doctor's office was full of portraits by Picasso.
—Rita Rudner

NO BOOK ON beauty would be complete without a chapter on cosmetic medicine. More than eleven million cosmetic surgical procedures were performed in the United States in 2006, according to the American Society for Aesthetic Plastic Surgery. It's a big deal, but if you think we're going to come down on one side or the other, think again. As with anything else involving health and beauty, it's not as simple as either saying, "Sure! Do it!" or wagging a finger in disapproval. These are personal decisions, and we won't be judgmental in any way.

First, an important distinction: we're going to talk about cosmetic medicine, but that doesn't mean only cosmetic surgery. It also means noninvasive procedures that can be done by a dermatologist. Our hope is that you will improve your inner and outer beauty as much as you can by the simplest, most holistic means possible from the beginning. For most women, aging may bring the desire for some noninvasive procedures, and that's fine.

The vast majority of the procedures are tested, safe, and effective. That said, we'll never condone a woman's neglecting her skin and mental health and trying to palliate problems by running to her dermatologist. That's like putting up wallpaper without first repairing the holes in the walls.

Unless you have a skin disease that requires medical treatment, this is the progression we suggest you follow to maximize your beauty:

- Care for your health, inner beauty, and outer beauty, and improve them as much as possible.
- If you still have beauty issues, talk to a dermatologist about noninvasive medicine.
- If some problems can't be resolved that way, you might consider a consultation with a plastic surgeon to discuss cosmetic surgery.

It's like everything else in *The Beauty Prescription*: you're responsible for your beauty. Start with healthy habits and affirming behaviors.

UNDER THE KNIFE FOR THE RIGHT REASONS

We're not opposed to cosmetic enhancement. It has been clearly shown to enhance people's quality of life. Extensive studies have documented that cosmetic treatments such as Botox and fillers really do make people feel remarkably better, improving self-esteem, creating healthier self-perception, and reducing anxiety over appearance.

Plastic surgery became popular in this country after World War I, when many soldiers came home with facial injuries that required reconstructive surgery. Development of these techniques helped launch the specialty that became elective cosmetic surgery—surgery that you undergo because you want to look better.

When considering cosmetic surgery, always weigh the potential benefits against the risks and costs (elective cosmetic surgery is not covered by insurance and can cost thousands of dollars) and decide if surgical intervention is really necessary. Are you considering it for the right reasons? Make sure you're thinking about it from a healthy perspective. Here's what we mean:

• **Healthy:** Through exercise and diet, you've gotten yourself very healthy, and as a result of your doing what you love, focusing on gratitude and compassion, and being optimistic, your inner beauty is shining. You feel that you're almost complete, but you'd like to have a little work done, to correct an issue that has been nagging at you and partially as a reward for all the other nurturing things you've done for yourself. You're done nursing your children, you're fit and healthy, and you would like breast augmentation.

• **Unhealthy:** Your marriage is in trouble, and you're blaming yourself because you don't look as perfect as you did when you were thirty. You're desperate to keep things together, because deep down, you don't believe anyone else would want you. You want breast augmentation as a last-ditch effort to save your relationship.

Not a lot of commentary needed, is there?

LOOK BETTER OR BE DIFFERENT?

If you're contemplating any kind of cosmetic medicine, ask yourself what you're trying to achieve. Do you want to look better because you feel you deserve to look and feel your best? That's a healthy motivation that comes from a place of self-love and confidence. In such cases, even some simple cosmetic work can be a real blessing. We have known women who, upon having a few injections of dermal filler such as Juvéderm to reduce and soften facial lines, broke into tears because they were so relieved to see that they could still look beautiful. From a healthy perspective, cosmetic medicine is like the final touch to you, the masterpiece.

It's one thing to want to look better. We all want that, and the self-esteem kick that accompanies it is a wonderful side effect. It's another matter to want cosmetic surgery so you can become, in effect, a different person. Cosmetic surgery is a deeply personal decision, and you should never have it because somebody else—a relative, husband, or employer—is pushing you to do it. Also, if you feel that you need to take such a drastic step, ask yourself, is it really because it will make someone else happier, or is that a rationalization? One large U.S. study revealed that 70 percent of married men thought their wives' breast size was just fine, yet many women assert that they have breast enlargements to please their mates. Who's telling the truth?

No cosmetic procedure will change who you are. All it will do is perhaps bring you closer to some innate beauty ideal that you carry in your head. Changing who you are is the province of evolving beauty, and it starts within, with your behaviors and attitudes. That's why it's vital to be clear about your expectations from any cosmetic medicine. Realistic expectations help match women to the proper procedure and provider. You should always be well informed about the procedure itself, what outcome you can expect, and the risks. Most of all, know what the procedure can do and what it can't do.

Women with unrealistic expectations—this surgery will get me the job, save my marriage, make my parents proud of me—inevitably end up disappointed. We know a woman who had extra fat removed from her thighs so she would look better in a bathing suit, but when the work was done, she still hated the way she looked. The problem was not in her thighs but in her self-image. Women with more realistic expectations will usually have a better experience with any form of cosmetic medicine. If you doubt your motivations or you're conflicted about wanting cosmetic surgery, it's a good idea to speak with a therapist to get an objective opinion.

FORGET DIAMONDS—RHINOPLASTY IS FOREVER

Many surgeries can be done once and yield a lifetime of improved appearance. For example, many women in their late teens or early twenties will opt to have rhinoplasty—a nose job—and will enjoy a more attractive face for the rest of their days. This is one of the most common surgeries, and we have seen it work wonders on women's self-esteem. Breast augmentation is also common for women who find themselves neck-deep in the dating pool or who are coming off multiple pregnancies and breast-feeding. Face-lifts, although still popular, may decline in the future with the rise of noninvasive procedures that can provide many of the same benefits.

The central point is that cosmetic surgery is a lifelong change. This is not something that should be entered into lightly. The best way to approach it is to do your research into procedures, risks, and physicians in your area who provide the services you want. Then scrutinize your motivation. If you're unsure, talk to a therapist who has experience in dealing with concerns related to cosmetic surgery. Then if you still decide to go ahead, adopt a positive mental attitude, and you can proceed knowing that the vast majority of women who undergo these procedures do look and feel better.

In fact, plastic surgery can change lives. A terrific example of this transformative power comes from a Malibu, California, woman in her forties whom we'll call Melinda. When she was fourteen, she was experiencing problem periods and was diagnosed with ovarian cysts. At fifteen, she went in for surgery, and the surgeons either nicked her uterus and were forced to remove it, or removed it accidentally. She never found out. Either way, it was a crushing blow. "You wake up at fifteen and find out you're never going to have children," she says.

She received help for the severe emotional trauma of the experience through therapy, but the physical legacy remained. The surgeon had left a large, puckered line of scar tissue over most of her abdomen, a visible reminder of her violation. The impact of this disfigurement was profound. At one point, she developed anorexia nervosa and at five feet tall was down to sixty-five pounds. "The hospital called my parents once to tell them I wasn't going to make it because my liver was shutting down," she recalls.

She recovered, but a lasting effect of her unattractive scar was to make her retreat from showing her body. She was and is a fit, slender woman, but every time she looked in the mirror, the scar was all she saw. "I carried that scar around like a war wound," she says. Until three years ago, she had never worn a two-piece bathing suit.

Three years ago, Melinda had abdominoplasty, also known as a "tummy tuck." The scar is now invisible below her bikini line, and she maintains that getting rid of her scar has changed

---

BEAUTY STORY: "CHARLOTTE"

Charlotte, thirty-two, came to see Debra for a consultation on treating some facial scarring. She was evasive when asked about the source of the scars, even though they were not serious enough to require a full-face laser resurfacing and could be treated with injectables. Debra was suspicious about her behavior, and after the treatment was finished and Charlotte was still highly self-critical about her appearance, Debra asked her if she was ready to share the source of her scarring. Charlotte then confided that they resulted from beatings by an ex-boyfriend. Debra immediately recommended that Charlotte seek the help of a therapist, whom she continues to see to this day.

Eva: You treated Charlotte's external scars, but she was concealing feelings of guilt regarding the terrible ordeal she had suffered. Battered women sometimes find themselves feeling guilty not only for testifying against the man who abused them but also for allowing themselves to be abused.

Debra: It was pretty obvious to me once she came back in a few months after the Restylane filler treatment that she was looking in the mirror and seeing something no one else could see. On the surface, Charlotte was an attractive woman—tall, athletic, striking if not classically beautiful—but her experience had twisted her self-perception, and nothing external was really going to change that.

her life in every way. "It was the first time I didn't feel raped or marred when I looked in the mirror," she says. "There's a difference in how I carry myself, in how I wear my makeup. That plastic surgery was absolutely life altering."

Melinda concludes: "This was the best gift I could ever have had, that I could feel not even beautiful but just normal. That I could wear a bathing suit or bikini underpants was normal and beautiful. You can have all the therapy in the world—and before one looks at serious surgery, one should have that—but that would never have done what the surgery did for me. It gave me my soul back. I look in the mirror and don't see what they did to me; I see a woman who has a beautiful body. Nothing else would have given me that, but the surgery did."

In Your Dermatologist's Office

Because neither of us is a plastic surgeon, we are going to discuss only procedures that do not require general anesthesia. These are noninvasive cosmetic procedures that can do much to address many if not all facial or skin concerns.

We're going to do this from the perspective of a patient's visit with a dermatologist. First, the dermatologist will examine your skin to see what problems or potential diseases exist. She'll be looking for abnormalities in skin pigmentation, broken capillaries, and anything that could be a precursor to skin cancer. This is why you should choose a doctor who is not just looking at the cosmetic aspect of your skin. If there's a skin cancer there, you want a doctor who's going to pay attention, not just laser over it.

The dermatologist may then hold up a mirror and examine your skin with you, asking you what you see and what particular aspects you would like to change. Then she will tell you what her practiced eye sees. If she notices abnormal growths, the first priority will be having a biopsy to determine if there's any cancer. This is not a cause for panic; if caught early, the most common forms of skin cancer are almost completely curable.

If there isn't any potential cancer, then the question will be: What do you want to do? This is where the Internet has become both blessing and curse—blessing because patients are coming to their cosmetic consultations more informed than ever; curse because, well, for the same reason. Some women walk in ready to tell the doctor what to do, demanding a certain procedure or product, perhaps because they've heard about it in the news. It's important to come into this consultation knowing what the different procedures are all about, but it's equally important to trust your dermatologist to use her expertise to design a cosmetic regimen that meets your needs. You should be working together.

Noninvasive Procedures

So, there's nothing that looks like cancer. You breathe a sigh of relief, and then your dermatologist tells you she sees plenty of signs of sun damage: brown spots, broken vessels, fine lines, and wrinkles. At this point, a good doctor will talk to you about a home skin-care regimen that can prevent further damage and also give you better results from your cosmetic procedures. Then you'll chat about resurfacing or rejuvenating the skin, from the lowest-intensity treatments to the most intense.

AT-HOME PROCEDURES. At the lowest rung of the ladder are the home glycolic peels or home chemical peels. These stay on the skin for anywhere from one minute to fifteen minutes, depending on the kind of acid in the peel and the severity of the problem. Significant changes will need at least four peels, spaced two to four weeks apart, to give your skin time to renew and heal.

IN-OFFICE PROCEDURES, MODERATE INTENSITY. Next up are in-office chemical peels using stronger solutions of glycolic, salicylic, or trichloroacetic acid. Microdermabrasion is another method to rejuvenate skin. Because doing this improperly at home can tear the skin, it's safer to have microdermabrasion done in an office setting, where a small vacuum sucks away excess crystals and skin cells. There is also a newer procedure, called dermal infusion microdermabrasion. One brand, Silk Peel, uses a diamond head to exfoliate the skin and can also infuse active boosters into the skin to help with pigmentation problems and acne.

IN-OFFICE PROCEDURES, HIGHER INTENSITY. Next on the intensity scale is intense pulse light treatment, or IPL, also called photorejuvenation. These are not lasers. Going by brand names such as Aurora and Quantum, they use a powerful light source to absorb abnormal blood vessels and pigmentation and tighten pores. Pore size is a frequent concern for patients, when in fact pores are a normal part of the hair follicle–sebaceous unit.

The next step up from IPL are the minimally ablative lasers. These include the erbium laser, or Laser Peel. These lasers require repeat treatments for maximal results. They improve pigmentation, fine lines, and acne scars. Even better, it takes only two to five days for redness and swelling to dissipate. Fractionated lasers such as the Fraxel laser are another option for treating pigmentation, fine lines, and acne scars. These lasers produce microcolumns of ablation into the skin and also require usually four to five treatments for maximal results with little downtime. The older ablative CO_2 laser is still valuable for treating severely sun-damaged and wrinkled skin, but it requires at least two weeks of healing time. The ablative lasers affect the under layers of the skin, stimulating collagen growth and treating wrinkles and hyperpigmentation.

One warning about lasers: Many new ones are coming into the market, and they carry the cachet of any new technology, but that doesn't mean every laser is right for you. The newest procedure isn't necessarily the best. Some new technologies have unpleasant side effects, and it may take a few years of fine-tuning before they can be made relatively comfortable for patients while remaining effective. Know what you're getting, and don't insist on the newest laser just because it's new.

As we age, our skin starts to sag. This sagging is not due to gravity; it results from changes in the collagen and elastin fibers in the skin. One noninvasive treatment to combat this problem is radio-frequency, or RF, therapy. An example of this technology is Thermage. This device uses radio waves to penetrate the skin deeply and heat the underlying collagen, causing it to contract and stimulate collagen production. This produces a subtle face-lift effect that's ideal for sagging brows, cheeks, and neck. Eyelids, arms, the abdomen, and legs can also be treated with this technology.

Sun Damage, Acne, and Rosacea. For individuals with recurrent precancers and sun damage, photodynamic therapy may be the most appropriate treatment. For this procedure, the doctor applies a medication called Levulin and then uses an intense pulse light or specialized laser on the area to be treated. This allows some abnormal cells to fade away while improving the appearance of fine lines, pigmentation, and broken capillaries, shrinking sebaceous glands and pores, and revitalizing collagen production.

For acne, the dermatologist may recommend a skin-care regimen along with various cosmetic procedures. Chemical peels, microdermabrasion, IPL, and treatments including blue light or acne lasers (examples: smooth beam and clear light) can be effective in the treatment and clearing of acne.

Finally, rosacea, or adult acne, is a common problem among fair-skinned individuals. Along with topical and oral prescription treatments including Metrogel, Finacea, and Oracea, there are effective in-office procedures for this problem, including glycolic peels and IPL treatments.

Lines Are for Movie Theaters

Not every person is a good candidate for every procedure. Women with rosacea, for instance, should not have microdermabrasion, because it can worsen outbreaks. Women with certain pigmentation types are also not good fits with some procedures, especially lasers that target specific areas of pigmentation and can leave darker-skinned women with light or dark spots. Again, talk to your doctor, and know what you're getting into.

Back to our fictional office consult. Let's say the sun damage isn't bad and acne isn't a problem. Now your dermatologist is going to look for contour changes: deeper lines around your nose, "marionette" lines that run from under your nose to your chin, forehead lines, frown lines, crow's-feet, and more. Once she identifies your lines, she'll devise treatment recommendations by dividing your face into three zones:

- Upper, from your upper brow to your nasal ridge
- Middle, from your nasal ridge to your upper lip
- Lower, from your upper lip to your chin

Upper-face wrinkles are usually *dynamic* wrinkles. As explained previously, they are called this not because they have a great personality but because they are caused by muscle movement. These lines may get a visit from a treatment that's so famous that it's become a synonym for cosmetic medicine:

BEAUTY BOOSTERS

Practical things you can do now to be more beautiful

Keep objects clean and free of microorganisms in your beauty space. Grooming products can be a free-for-all for bacteria. Clean or toss old loofahs and other shower items. Use your hands to wash your face and body. Throw away makeup more than three months old. Wash your face every night to remove your makeup. Change your razor with every other use, and never store it in the shower; showers are breeding grounds for bacteria, fungi, and viral warts. Wash your pillowcase weekly (at least) with a nonperfumed detergent.

Precautions such as these will help you avoid bacterial infections, prevent fungal infections such as those that can damage your nails, keep your makeup doing its job, and keep your beauty space smelling clean and fresh.

Botox. Botox uses a modified version of botulinum toxin to relax facial muscles and smooth wrinkles.

With this popular treatment come some warnings. Certain patients cannot have Botox, such as people with neuromuscular disease. Also, be careful about unlicensed practitioners administering Botox. Performing this procedure can be lucrative, and we're constantly hearing horror stories about doctors with little or no dermatological training and even salons doing Botox, sometimes with highly negative results such as severe reactions.

Next come the eyes, a particularly sensitive area both because the skin is delicate and because your eyes have so much to do with how others perceive your appearance. Procedures such as Thermage can be performed to tighten the eyelids. Hyaluronic fillers such as Restylane can also be injected into the hollows or tear troughs around the eyes to make the eyes look less sunken or sallow. Cosmoderm, a fine-line filler, can soften crow's-feet, as can Botox. Sometimes, the two products can be used together in this area. You can also consider blepharoplasty, or an eyelid lift, but you'll need to consult a cosmetic or oculoplastic surgeon.

THE MIDDLE AND LOWER FACE. We come now to the proud bow of the female face, the noble nose. A dermatologist can do some reshaping of the nose with injectables, and these can last usually six to nine months. However, a new nose usually means rhinoplasty (a nose job), and that means surgery.

Moving down to the lower third of the face, we find the aforementioned nasolabial lines running from the nose to the corners of the mouth and "marionette" lines that run from the mouth to the chin. Injectable fillers are life changers here. You have a wide variety from which to choose. Long-lasting fillers include Perlane, Juvederm, Cosmoderm, Cosmoplast, Restylane, Sculptra, and Radiesse. You can even have your own body fat siphoned off and used as a filler, sort of a personal form of recycling. Fillers are a popular procedure because they show immediate results, are relatively painless, and have few side effects. However, beware of permanent fillers, because as you age, your skin drapes differently, and you don't want to be trading a wrinkle for a ridge. Permanent fillers include Artefill and silicone; ask your physician if these are appropriate for you.

"In addition to wrinkles in the middle and lower face, volume loss appears in these areas as we age," notes Florida cosmetic dermatologist Mark Nestor, M.D., Ph.D., president of the International Society of Cosmetic and Laser Surgeons. "The face is like a deflating balloon, and often the best treatment is filling these areas up, or 'volumizing.' Hyaluronic fillers or fat transfer is usually the best option for treatment."

Moving south to the lips, we notice that they shrink as collagen breaks down and is not renewed. Of the many lip rejuvenation techniques, the most popular involve the injection of fillers such as hyaluronic acid, sometimes combining these with fine-line fillers such as Cosmoderm. Surgeons can also use lip implants or can surgically correct for a more permanent effect.

Now we come to the neck, chin, and jawline. This is where many women will notice sagging skin as they age. Radiofrequency procedures such as Thermage are an excellent treatment for sagging skin in these areas. These procedures cause some immediate tightening and then continual tightening during the following six months or so as new collagen forms, making the skin firmer. These results usually last between two and three years. Another option is infrared (IR) treatment under brand names such as Skin-Tyte and Titan. These machines use IR energy to penetrate and heat the skin and remodel collagen.

Hair Today, Gone Tomorrow

Hair-related problems are another area in which your dermatologist can help. Among women in or past menopause, thinning hair is a fairly common problem. Stress, medication, and hormonal changes can cause hair to fall out. The first step is to discover if the hair loss has a medical cause such as a thyroid condition, anemia, or an autoimmune disease. If it's genetic female-pattern baldness (yes, there is such a thing), then there are other options. Biotin supplements are one; over-the-counter or prescription Rogaine is another. There's even a laser comb that women can use twice a day to stimulate hair growth, and as a last resort, there's hair transplantation.

On the other end of the spectrum we have women with too much hair, a condition called hirsutism. For routine hair removal, there are numerous treatment options, including shaving, waxing, depilatories, electrolysis, and threading. For permanent hair reduction, lasers or IPL are the preferred choices. However, as stated previously, lasers are not suitable for every skin type. They tend to work best for people who have fair skin but dark hair. Dark-skinned individuals need to approach laser treatments with caution, because as the laser goes after the pigment in the hair follicle and destroys it, it can accidentally take the pigment out of the skin. So, you should never get laser hair removal when you're tan or even using a self-tanning lotion.

There is also an intense pulse light treatment that can be used for people with somewhat dark skin, such as Asian and Hispanic women. If you're fortunate, you can experience what's called permanent reduction of excess hair: 80 percent of the hairs may be gone for good, but you come back two or three times per year for treatments to take care of the remaining 20 percent that doesn't take the hint.

Spiders, Cottage Cheese, and Saddlebags, Oh My!

Our tour winds up with a few conditions that don't affect the face but are of particular interest to women: spider veins, cellu-

---

BEAUTY PEARLS

A woman's sense of her own beauty should be giving to the environment, not taking from it. If you walk into Versailles, why would you think it's making you feel beautiful? You would be thinking how beautiful Versailles is.

Lighting is the most important thing a woman can change to make her surroundings more conducive to beauty. Make sure your lampshades throw a flattering glow. Create lighting you'd want to be photographed in. After that, make sure you don't have any what I call "monster mirrors" around. We all know what they are. Certain mirrors that for some reason make you look and feel tired, hideous, and older. All mirrors are NOT the same. If you've got any harsh mirrors, reposition them in some dark basement, donate them to a men's room somewhere, or get rid of them.

Finally, the simplest way to make a woman's environment more beauty-conducive is to clear it out. Prune your physical surroundings of clutter. If you can't do it yourself, seek professional help because creating a clear, clean environment is the best way to achieve serenity, the most beauty-conducive condition in the world.

—Kathryn Ireland, textile designer

lite, and excess fat. Spider veins are caused by blood backing up into the tiny vessels of the legs. Varicose veins are caused by the same process, but they are larger and can lead to blood clots or phlebitis, so women with varicose veins should consult a vascular surgeon. There are several advanced treatments for spider veins, such as lasers and radio frequency. These are often helpful, but for some people, they don't appear to work as well as an old-fashioned approach: sclerotherapy. Here a doctor injects a solution into the affected vein that causes it to shut off from blood flow. Eventually, with two to ten treatments, the vein dissolves.

Then there is cellulite, the bane of thighs and buttocks everywhere. We hate to break it to you, but those dimples below the waist are perfectly normal and natural. They are not fat, and they are not a disease. They are caused by the fibrous bands that form between fat globules. Plenty of topical products, machines, and skin massagers have been touted as cures for cellulite. Some, such as the nonsurgical procedures Endermologie (a kind of skin vacuum) or Velasmooth or Triactive (both laser treatments), can provide a temporary benefit, but none will do the job permanently. If you are bothered by cellulite, your best bet for minimizing it is eating a good diet and keeping your muscles and skin toned and firm with exercise. Then forget about cellulite and focus on things that you can do something about.

Combating excess fat in the abdomen, thighs, and waist can seem like a never-ending battle. Many women have tried every imaginable exercise to reduce these areas, but to no avail. These areas of excess fat often are the product of genetic or hormonal factors. There is a minimally invasive procedure that can help, however. Called tumescent liposuction, it uses local anesthesia and saline water to numb the skin and fat. The fat is then removed using microcannulas, small strawlike tubes, to contour these areas with minimal risk. Newer adjuvant treatments such as Smart Lipo can give additional benefit in fat contouring. Liposuction, let's be clear, is not a weight-loss technique. It is an appropriate alternative for patients within twenty pounds of their ideal body weight who want to contour areas of excess fat.

CHOOSING YOUR PLASTIC SURGEON

The TV series "Nip/Tuck" makes plastic surgery look deviant and dangerous. When performed by a skilled, board-certified surgeon, it's anything but. Millions of women have cosmetic procedures performed every year, and the large majority have few complications and are happy with the results. That said, we

---

     BEAUTY BUSTERS

Beauty myths debunked while you wait

Myth: Cosmetic surgery always looks unnatural.
Fact: These days, it seems as if everyone is walking around with fish lips and no facial expression, especially in our necks of the woods—Beverly Hills and South Beach. Those are almost always cases of overdone collagen and Botox, not botched plastic surgery. There are thousands of cosmetic practitioners among us, and a certain percentage are poorly trained in aesthetics or proper technique. What you might not know is that many attractive women are walking around with properly applied Botox and collagen, but you would never guess they had these procedures. That is the "no telltale" sign of a good cosmetic practitioner.

hope you will take any decisions concerning plastic surgery and anesthesia seriously.

Surgery may be common, but it always carries risks. Do your homework. Consult with at least three surgeons. Ask to see photos of their work. Some people even choose to interview the potential anesthesiologist. Check to see if prospective providers are board certified. Make sure the surgical facility is certified. Talk to other women who have had procedures performed by the surgeon, and check their credentials on the Internet (see the Resources for websites where you can do this). Whatever you do, don't make a decision based on price. We are talking about your body and life here, not the latest designer jeans.

With all these options comes a simple bit of wisdom: buyer, beware. We have seen women become so excited about the potential of cosmetic medicine to enhance their outer beauty and their lives that they leave their critical-thinking skills on the bedside table. As you explore these promising ways to further become the most beautiful you possible, be sure to ask plenty of questions, and take grandiose claims with a grain of salt.

For informed help in choosing your doctor, ask for a referral from your family physician or ob-gyn, or from a woman you know who has been happy with her cosmetic medicine experience. A few further cautions:

- Choose a doctor who has a lot of experience performing the treatment in which you're interested but who is conservative about using new technologies and isn't going to jump on the bandwagon of a new machine just because it's new.
- Choose someone board-certified in dermatology or plastic surgery. Look for certification from the American Board of Dermatologists or the American Board of Plastic Surgery.

- Look for a well-trained aesthetician—a skin-care specialist who can work in concert with your dermatologist in offering you professional care. We prefer to recommend aestheticians who have some medical training or who work out of a medical office, so that a physician is on hand to supervise the work. Aestheticians are good at educating patients about skin care, helping them work with skin-care routines, and even doing procedures such as mild peels, microdermabrasion, and facials. Whatever you are having done, always check out your aesthetician's licensing and education, as requirements vary by state.
- Try to find a beauty team: a physician, a nurse-practitioner or physician's assistant, and an aesthetician who can work together for the benefit of your skin.
- Try to find a doctor who is doing clinical trials and research. Such doctors likely will be up on the latest literature and advances in the field.
- Don't ask your doctor for specific treatments. Talk about the specific problems you want to address, and let your doctor come up with a medically reliable plan.

Cosmetic medicine can be a real asset not just for your outer beauty but for your quest for greater inner beauty as well.

Beauty Bullets

ᐵ Cosmetic medicine is wonderful when it's consumed wisely.

ᐵ Focus on your health and well-being first, and then consider cosmetic medicine to address issues that holistic methods cannot.

ᕲ Always know your motivations for wanting cosmetic intervention.

ᕲ Cosmetic procedures are a personal choice; never feel pressured to have a procedure. It's not for everyone.

ᕲ A vast range of noninvasive cosmetic procedures can address sun damage, wrinkles, and thinning and excess hair.

ᕲ Cellulite is natural, and there aren't any truly effective treatments for it.

ᕲ Choose your physician with care, and ask questions.

 ## BEAUTY AND THE BRAIN Rx

An Ounce of Prevention

Dr. Debra: *If you want a tan, do what Charlize Theron did for the 2004 Oscars: use the faux stuff. Since you are not going to sit in the sun again without UV protection (right?), you'll save your money, avoid tanning salons, and still look bronzed without the risk or the price tag. The new self-tanners and bronzers have come a long way. Self-tanners come in all kinds of applications: towels, foams, sprays, and lotions. Go ahead and experiment. There are even salons that will apply the self-tan for you.*

The dermatologist's secret to a better self-tan? Exfoliate first, getting rid of the dead skin cells. After applying the tanning product, wait for the solution to dry before engaging in any activity. Also, wash your hands following application so you don't have tan palms. You can even choose a self-tanner or bronzer with a built-in SPF, so you get two for the price of one.

Dr. Eva: *Start trying to notice patterns of thinking or behavior that you've fallen into. We all succumb to unconscious patterns, some of which are benign, such as driving a certain route to work. Other patterns, though, are harmful, such as constantly berating ourselves for physical imperfections or being overly self-critical. Think about the times that you have tried to make changes in your behavior. How successful were you? Why did you fail? Becoming aware of self-defeating patterns of behavior is the first step to lasting change. Let's say you want to lose weight but have failed every time in the past. Did you sabotage your healthy eating habits? Why? What can you do this time around to change that? Be alert to specific patterns over a period of days or weeks, and note how they impact your inner and outer beauty. When you are aware of patterns that are harmful, you can take steps to alter them and stop making the same mistakes.*

11

Wearing Pearls with Scrubs

The future belongs to those who believe in the beauty of their dreams.

—Eleanor Roosevelt

SINCE WE MET in medical school at Tufts University, in Boston, our lives have been filled with amazing coincidences that seem to defy explanation. In fact, until we ended up practicing on opposite coasts, we were pretty much inseparable. Today, we are fortunate to spend so much time together on the phone or online that sometimes we forget that we live three thousand miles apart. Writing this book together has given us the opportunity to literally finish each other's sentences.

When we were doing our internships in Los Angeles—a scene right out of "Grey's Anatomy," all crazy schedules and no sleep—we did our utmost to maintain our femininity, individuality, and sanity while working thirty-six-hour shifts. One of the easy chores that year was figuring out what to wear. Not too much choice in that department. Donning the obligatory green doctors' scrubs every day cut way down on time spent in the closet and on money spent at the dry cleaner or mall. Even so, we tried to look our best, and at twenty-something it was a much easier task. Debra's husband, who is an ER doctor, was drawn to her because she looked cute in scrubs. We will never forget the original "beauty buddies" outing when he sent us off for a day at the spa before exams.

Eva's husband always says that he decided to ask her out because "she was the only one wearing pearls with her scrubs." He went on to become a cosmetic dermatologist, keeping the girlfriend synchronicity alive and well. Many years have elapsed since then, but our philosophy remains the same: being as beautiful as you can be, inside and out, makes good things happen in your life. Friendships, giving and finding beauty in the most unusual places or times, is what it's all about.

So, this chapter offers a few final thoughts—no sidebars, no tips; just girlfriends sharing a few "pearls" with you.

A BEAUTIFUL OUTLOOK ON LIFE

Okinawans are among the longest-lived people on Earth. Gerontologists suspect one of the reasons for this is that they cultivate long-lasting social circles, called *yuimaru*. On the island, friends and relatives come together regularly to support each other, laugh, and share life's experiences. They care for one another during illness and bereavement. In this way, they are much like women all over the world. We draw resiliency, energy, and optimism from coming together in groups.

Reach out and build your own yuimaru. Women are wonderful at creating support networks that are godsends during good times as well as more challenging times. Being together, sharing common experiences and laughing, is essential—physically, emotionally, and spiritually. Friendship is a vital and invigorating part of a beautiful life.

REACH FOR THE STARRS

Starr Sariego is someone who is truly working the Beauty-Brain Loop. Starr (what a perfect name!) is genetically blessed—tall and slender, with green eyes and brown hair. She's also exceptionally happy with the life she has created. In her twenties, she worked as a flight attendant, which gave her the opportunity to see the world. When she married and had children, she gave up flying to stay home and take care of her family. She never regretted the decision and has relished the time with her kids and husband. Now that her children are older, she has found the time to start a business locating beautiful homes for modeling photo shoots. It's flexible and fulfilling and lets her keep family at the center of her life.

Starr has that unique blend of perspective and gratitude that makes every part of life glow with joy. At fifty, she's had her share of adversity—she lost a sister to cancer—but that hasn't turned her outlook on life negative. On the contrary, it's made her appreciate her blessings more. Starr has all the aspects of the loop kicked into high gear. Her inner beauty is shining with a positive outlook and gratitude for all the blessings in her life.

"Out of most of my friends, I think I'm the happiest with my life," she says. "Sure, you can always want more, like more money, kids with no adolescent problems, a perfect marriage, but the gift is in acknowledging life the way it is and loving it."

Starr's outer beauty shines as well. She gets facials regularly. She is always dressed attractively, showing her artistic side. She is at the gym most mornings. She is conscientious about maintaining her health and eats primarily an organic vegetarian diet. Her environment is also a reflection of her beauty. Her home is always filled with food, friends, and laughter. And she is always the first to help out in a crisis, large or small. Her method of coping with tough times? "Slow down when times are rough, and take comfort from friends," she says.

The core of Starr's beauty is loving herself inside and out. She doesn't mind the changes in her face as she ages. She says, "I think my face reflects my experiences, tells my story, and gives me character. I see the same with my girlfriends. It's what they project when they walk into a room, who they have become in the world, how they make other people feel. What I see in any person is the inner happiness that's reflected in her face." That is evolving beauty—the ability of your perception of beauty to grow and deepen—at its finest. For Starr, the future is always bright. We hope you will find someone like this to inspire you. We're lucky. We have a Starr to guide us.

CLEAR UP SKIN CARE

Another example of *The Beauty Prescription* spirit is Debi Byrnes. She had bad acne as a teenager and was so traumatized by it that she became a licensed skin-care professional to learn more about the disorder that left her with some serious psychological scars. Later, she wanted to help other teens avoid her experience, but there was one small problem: there was no established outlet.

"In 2002, I was thinking I would really like to volunteer at a place that taught skin care to teens," she says, "but I couldn't find anything in the United States. I had previously started a nonprofit organization for someone else, so I thought, 'OK, I'll just do it for myself.'" So, in 2004, ClearUpSkinCare.org was born. Today, during her free time, Debi visits health classes at two Greater Los Angeles middle schools and a high school to talk to students about acne—how to prevent it, treat it, and avoid having their self-esteem harmed by it.

"I teach the kids how to take care of their skin and how they can get their acne under control," she says, "but more important, I teach them that it's not the be-all and end-all of them, that they shouldn't let acne hold them back. When you have acne, you're self-conscious. You can feel as if you're not as good as other people. Young people tend to feel that they have to do more if they don't feel good about themselves, but if you love yourself, no matter what you look like, you're going to do great."

Talk about inner beauty! Debi has channeled her own trauma into something that could benefit thousands of teens. She continues to strive to meet new goals. "I would really like ClearUp SkinCare to be larger," she says, "with a psychologist leading groups for adults who have been scarred emotionally by acne. I've never seen anything like that. I think it would be wonderful for these adults to heal some of these wounds they had as adolescents." Debi's positive outlook inspires us to give back to those in need and is a reminder that life's challenges can become strengths.

STRINGING THE PEARLS TOGETHER

Women such as Starr, Debi, and the others we've featured in this book are living examples of what can happen when you commit to putting the Beauty-Brain Loop into action every day of your life. Before we complete this journey, let's take one more look at the loop:

- **Inner beauty:** It begins and ends with self-esteem, having realistic expectations for yourself and being forgiving when you don't live up to some kind of ideal. Inner beauty is about living in the moment, taking joy in life whenever you can, and learning to see beauty everywhere and in everyone. Relationships are essential, as is finding meaning in your life, wherever you find it. Inner beauty is evolving beauty, in which you see yourself as more complete and beautiful over time, and you develop the magnetism that makes you irresistible to others. If life's bumps don't get you down, you are sure to become a more beautiful woman as you grow and learn along life's journey.

- **Health:** Health is a gift, and it's up to you and no one else to take care of it. Health is beautiful, so go back to basics: eat well, exercise, sleep, give yourself times of peace and meditation, learn to shed stress the way a duck sheds water, and form a partnership with your doctor to care for your health. Women can and do live longer and healthier lives than ever before. Do it looking amazing!

- **Outer beauty:** We start with innate beauty, the kind that we're all programmed to perceive and desire. Society expects you to fit into a certain template, but that's society's problem. Your only duty is to be as beautiful as you want to be—and to be the kind of beautiful you want to be, whether that's formal European style or California beach casual. You are always a work in progress, so apart from taking lifelong care of your skin, hair, nails, and teeth, don't be afraid to step out and try something new and daring. Experiment. It doesn't matter how old you are. When you feel more beautiful, your inner beauty shines as well.

- **Environment:** Your relationships, home, career, social circles, and life's purpose are all part of your environment. This component of the loop is finding beauty, creating beauty, and sharing beauty. Live encircled by people who love you and whom you can love back. Teach others to recognize beauty in the everyday. Seek out pursuits that bring you joy and meaning.

Each area of the loop is like an individual pearl: when you string them together, their value and beauty multiplies.

BEAUTY IS A JOURNEY

To engage the loop and have it working for you inside and out and in your environment, you must commit to the actions and attitudes that evoke beauty in you and your world. Beauty isn't a destination; it's a journey. You don't arrive at a place and say, "All right, I'm gorgeous. Now what?" You should be growing, changing, and discovering every day of your life. In the end, beauty should become your *lifestyle*.

This means making the deliberate effort to work every stage of the loop as often as you can. Take care of your health daily; that's the most obvious one. Exercise, eat well—you know the rest. Just as important, be good to yourself. Be optimistic. Nurture your inner beauty. Do things that you care about, and grow your confidence the way you build your muscles at the gym. Care for your skin and your outer beauty as part of your daily routine. Bring beauty into your environment, whether it's redesigning your home or expressing your love and admiration to the family, friends, and colleagues in your life.

That's a lot to ask, but you've got something to help you along: this book. We hope you'll dog-ear the corners, make notes in the margins, tear out pages and stick them on the fridge, retake the quiz—whatever it takes to keep you moving in the right direction on your journey. This is only the beginning of our relationship; we're going to be around to help you evolve into the most beautiful woman you can be.

BEAUTY AND THE BEAST

You know the classic story of "Beauty and the Beast": a beautiful woman is held captive by a hideous beast who she discovers is actually kind and noble. Eventually, she falls in love with the creature, having seen his true inner beauty, and he becomes human again. In the end, his inner beauty and outer beauty are in synchrony as he is restored by her love. Our twist is a bit different. Rather than waiting for someone to discover your inner beauty, we hope that this book has led you to your best ally, your brain. It's up to each of us to find our own inner beauty. When we do, we too are magically transformed.

Coming from two separate medical specialties—beauty and the brain—we've come together to create a new way of looking at beauty and becoming more beautiful. We've tried to bring two facets of every woman—her inner beauty and outer beauty—together to form something completely unique: a fresh, holistic standard by which each woman can measure herself as she grows.

LAST WORD

Before we go back to our practices and our own beauty journeys, we have one thing to say: thanks!

Being a physician and caring for the health of others is always an honor; it's why we do what we do. We're equally honored and grateful that you've spent your valuable time with us and made it all the way to the end. Writing *The Beauty Prescription* has changed us by forcing us to examine our own feelings about our own beauty, and we realize that we're still evolving, too. We're taking more time to see the beauty in ourselves, each other, and the world around us. We appreciate the gift of every day.

To our amazement and delight, our parallel lives continue. We had our daughters six months apart. The first time we brought them together, they were wearing the same pajamas. We continue to celebrate life together, sharing milestones and traveling as a large extended family. We visit beautiful places together: Alaska, Jamaica, Scotland. We still enjoy our beauty breaks together, only now we take our daughters along to the nail salon. Our mothers have also become friends, and it turns out that they are cut from similar cloth—two intellectual, beautiful women who share the same values. They are connected and involved in their communities and with their families, and both are grandmothers extraordinaire. We feel fortunate and deeply grateful to have such beauty in our lives.

We're also indebted to you and to all the incredible women who have inspired us and continue to inspire us. We're all in this together, and the possibilities are endless. We're all partners in redefining what it means to be beautiful—and what it means to be a woman. We hope to leave the world a better place for all of our daughters.

Please visit us at thebeautyprescription.com to share your stories with us and tell us about your "beauty buddy." We also invite you to visit us at beautyandthebrain.com, where you can take our unique Beauty and the Brain Quiz and discover how balanced a beauty you are, as well as sign up for regular beauty tips and a lot more. We have so much to share with you, and we're just getting started.

Sit down on that park bench, take a deep breath, and see the beauty all around you. You're a part of it, too.

Shopping the Beauty Counter with Dr. Debra

Walking through the beauty department of any major department store is enough to make you dizzy. Hundreds of products by hundreds of companies all promise to make us look like Sienna Miller until we're ninety. But which ones are worth your money? Which ones are most effective? Come shopping with Dr. Debra, and she'll fill you in.

Back in Chapter 6, we defined many of these product categories, so you should have some idea of what they do. Others, such as eye cream, are obvious. This list gives you the brand-name products that Dr. Debra has found to be safe and effective, along with some idea of what they cost. Using this roster, you can create your own shopping list that fits your budget. A few other points:

* There's little difference in quality and value between products you buy at the department store and what you buy at the drugstore. The ingredients are generally the same, except when it comes to newer peptides or growth factors. Otherwise, the only difference is in the jars, which tend to be more elegant at a

department store, and the cost, which can be two or three times higher. Overall, the difference is, shall we say, cosmetic.

• The only items worth a splurge are the antioxidant and peptide delivery systems, because the best ones promote new collagen growth and cellular health.

• Look for a chemical-free sunblock or a broad-spectrum sunscreen with stabilizers such as Mexoryl or Helioplex and with a minimum SPF of 15 to 30. The FDA's new "four star" rating system uses a series of stars to indicate a sunscreen's UVA protection. Note that if you live in a region where the sun is more intense, such as the mountains or desert, you should use sunscreen with SPF 30 to 45.

You'll notice that there are no toners, scrubs, or adhesive strips on our list. Many toners are alcohol based and can irritate, strip, and dehydrate the skin, leaving it red, wrinkled, and overly dry. Scrubs not only can be irritating but also can cause microabrasions and broken capillaries. Adhesive strips can tear your skin and should be avoided.

As far as acne products are concerned, buy an acne system for comprehensive treatment for this condition. Acne systems should be simple to use; with compliance, they can deliver rewarding benefits.

Pricing System

$: less than $10

$$: between $10 and $24

$$$: between $25 and $49

$$$$: between $50 and $100

$$$$$: more than $100

Cleansers

Gentle

Aveeno Positively Radiant Cleanser	$
Cera Ve Cleanser	$
Cetaphil Cleanser	$
Dove Cool Moisture Foaming Cleanser	$
Kinerase Gentle Daily Cleanser	$$$
Neutrogena Gentle Cleanser	$
Pond's Cold Cream Deep Cleanser	$
Prada Purifying Milk/Face	$$$
Prescriptives All Cream Cleanser	$$
Purpose Gentle Cleansing Wash	$
Revalé Skin Facial Cleanser	$$$
Topix Resurfix Ultra Gentle Cleanser	$$

Exfoliative

Aqua Glycolic Cleanser by Merz	$$
DDF Glycolic Exfoliating Wash 7%	$$
Dior Prestige Cleansing Crème	$$$
Gly Derm Gentle Cleanser (with glycolic acid 2%)	$
Jan Marini Bioglycolic Facial Cleanser	$$
Kinerase Pro Therapy Skin Smoothing Cleanser	$$$
M.D. Forte Facial Cleanser II (with glycolic acid 15%/20%)	$$
NeoStrata Facial Cleanser	$$
Neutrogena Oil Free Acne Wash	$
Therapeutix/Clarity Clarifying Cleanser	$$
Topix Replenix Fortified Cleanser	$$

Sunscreens

SPF Alone

Aveeno Continuous Protection Sunblock Lotion SPF 30 or SPF 45	$
Dermalogica Solar Defense Booster SPF 30	$$
Neutrogena Sensitive Skin Sunblock Lotion SPF 30	$
Neutrogena Ultra Sheer Dry-Touch Sunblock with Helioplex SPF 70	$
SkinCeuticals Ultimate UV Defense SPF 30 (contains Z-Cote)	$$
Topix Glycolix Elite Sunscreen SPF 30	$$

Oil-Free Facial Sunscreen

Banana Boat SunWear Faces Oil-Free SPF 30	$$
Clarins UV Plus Protective Day Screen Oil-Free SPF 40	$
Colorescience SPF 30	$$$
Coppertone Oil Free Faces SPF 30	$
Neutrogena Ultra Sheer Dry-Touch Sunblock with Helioplex SPF 55	$$

SPF Moisturizer

Aveeno Positively Radiant Daily Moisturizer SPF 15	$
Cetaphil Daily Facial Moisturizer with SPF 15	$
Dove Energy Glow Facial Brightening Moisturizer with SPF 15	$
Elizabeth Arden Extreme Conditioning Cream SPF 15	$$
Eucerin Sensitive Facial Skin Extra Protective Moisture Lotion with SPF 30	$
Exuviance Essential Multi-Defense Day Crème SPF 15	$$
Lancôme UV Expert SPF20 with Mexoryl	$$$
L'Oréal Revitalift UV with Mexoryl SX	$$
Neutrogena Healthy Defense Daily Moisturizer SPF 45 with Helioplex	$
Olay Complete Defense Daily UV Moisturizer SPF 30	$
Purpose Dual Treatment Moisture Lotion with SPF 15	$

SPF Moisturizer and Antioxidant

Avon Hydrofirming Bio Day Cream SPF 15	$$
Elizabeth Arden First Defense Anti-Oxidant Cream SPF 15	$$
Estée Lauder Daywear Plus Multi Protection Anti-Oxidant Crème SPF 15 for Dry Skin	$$
Kinerase Cream with SPF 15/30	$$$$
La Roche-Posay Anthelios SX SPF 15 Cream	$$
Lancôme Renergie Intense Lift SPF 15	$$$
Prescriptives Insulation Anti-Oxidant Vitamin Cream SPF 15	$$

Non-SPF Moisturizer

Clinique Dramatically Different Moisturizing Lotion	$$$
Dove Pro-Age Rich Night Cream	$$
GlyDerm Hydrotone Lite Moisturizer	$$$
Kinerase Pro-Therapy Ultra Rich Night Repair	$$$$$
Lancôme Absolute Premium BX	$$$$$
L'Oréal Skin Genesis	$$
Neocutis Bio-Restorative	$$$$$
Shiseido Bio Performance Super Restoring Cream	$$$$

Home Peels

Avon Anew Clinical Retexturizing Peel	$$$
Kinerase Instant Radiance Facial Peel	$$$$
MD Skincare Alpha Beta Daily Face Peel	$$$$
Philosophy The MicroDelivery Peel	$$$$
RoC Resurfacing Facial Peel Kit	$$$

Antioxidants

Care by Stella McCartney Radiance + Youth Elixir	$$$
Eucerin CoQ10 Anti-Wrinkle Cream	$$

Kinerase Pro Therapy Cream	$$$$$
La Roche-Posay Active C Light	$$$
Neutrogena Healthy Skin Anti-Wrinkle Lotion	$$
Origins A Perfect World White Tea Skin Guardian	$$$
Prevage MD	$$$$$
Revaléskin Night Cream	$$$$$
SkinCeuticals C E Ferulic	$$$
SkinCeuticals Phyto Corrective Gel	$$$

Home Microdermabrasion

Estée Lauder Idealist Micro-D Deep Thermal Refinisher	$$
L'Oréal ReFinish Micro-Dermabrasion Kit	$
Prada Hydrating Cream/Face	$$$

Peptide Creams

Dr. Brandt R3P Cream	$$$$$
Freeze 24/7 Icecream AntiAging Moisturizer	$$$$
Kinerase C6 Peptide	$$$$$
Olay Regenerist Micro-Sculpting Cream*	$$$
Peter Thomas Roth Unwrinkle	$$$$$
Reclaim with Argireline Revolutionary Nightime Anti-Aging Cream	$$$
Therapeutix Care and Repair SPF 15	$$$

Growth Factor

Citrix CRS 20% Serum with Growth Factors	$$$$
Jan Marini Transformation Cream	$$$$$
PCA Skin (pHaze 24) Rejuvenating Serum	$$$

*Olay Regenerist is an inexpensive cream that was compared during testing to more expensive creams by the Good Housekeeping Research Institute.

TNS Recovery Complex	$$$$$
Triax Pyratine-6	$$$$

Retinols

Afirm 1X/2X/3X Cream	$$$
Avene Retrinal	$$$$
Estée Lauder Diminish Anti-Wrinkle Treatment	$$$
La Roche-Posay Biomedic Retinol Cream	$$$
Natural Advantage Natural Renewal Complex	$$$
Neutrogena Healthy Skin Antiwrinkle Anti-Blemish Clear Skin Cream	$$
Neutrogena Healthy Skin Visibly Even Night Concentrate	$$
Philosophy Help Me Face Cream	$$
Replenix Retinol Smoothing Serum by Topix	$$$
RoC Retinol Actif Pur	$$$
Topix Replenix Retinol Smoothing Serum 5X	$$

Eye Creams

Aveeno Positively Radiant Eye Brightening Cream	$$
Chanel Precision Sublimage Eye Essential Regenerating Eye Cream	$$$$$
Elizabeth Arden Prevage Anti Aging Eye Treatment	$$
Estée Lauder Future Perfect	$$$
GlyDerm Hydrating Eye Cream	$$
La Prairie Cellular Eye Moisturizer	$$$
MD Skincare Lift & Lighten Eye Cream	$$
Neutrogena Radiance Boost Eye Cream	$
Neutrogena Visibly Firm Eye Cream	$
Nivea Visage Coenzyme Q10 Plus Wrinkle Control Eye Cream with SPF 4	$

Olay Age Defying Revitalizing Eye Gel	$$
Olay Definity Eye Illuminator	$$$
Peter Thomas Roth AHA/Kojic Under Eye Brightener	$$
Pond's Age DefEYE Eye Therapy	$
SkinCeuticals Eye Balm	$$$

Self-Tanners

Clarins Radiance-Plus Self Tanning Cream-Gel	$$
Dior Golden Self-Tanner	$$$
Estée Lauder Go Bronze Plus	$$
Estée Lauder Go Tan Sunless Towelettes	$$$
Neutrogena Build a Tan	$
Neutrogena Instant Bronze Streak-Free Foam	$
Origins Faux Glow Self-Tanner	$$
Philosophy The Healthy Tan	$

Acne Treatments

Acne Systems

Clean and Clear Advantage Acne Control Kit	$$
Clinique Acne Solutions	$$$
Neutrogena with Benzoyl Peroxide, Advanced Solutions Complete Acne Therapy System	$$$
Therapeutix System	$$$$

Acne Spot Therapy

Clearasil Ultra Vanishing Acne Treatment Cream	$
Good Skin All Right Spot Treatment	$
Kinerase Clear Skin Blemish Dissolver	$$$
MD Skincare Correct & Perfect Spot Treatment	$$
Therapeutix Emergency Outbreak Stick	$$

Acne Masks

Kinerase Clear Skin Regulating Mask	$$$$
Neutrogena Blackhead Eliminating Treatment Mask	$
Peter Thomas Roth Sulfur Cooling Mask	$$$

Rosacea/Redness Treatments

Aveeno Ultra Calming Moisturizing Cream	$
Avene Diroseal	$$$$
B. Kamins Booster Blue Rosacea Treatment	$$$
Clinique Redness Solutions Daily Relief Cream	$$$
Eucerin Redness Relief Night Cream	$$
La Roche-Posay Skin Perfecting Anti-Redness Moisturizer	$$$
Therapeutix System	$$$$
Weil For Origins Mega-Mushroom Face Cream	$$$

Brown Spot Treatments

Cellex-C Fade Away Gel	$$$$
Clarins Bright Plus On-the-Spot Brightening Corrector	$$$$
IS Clinical Active Serum	$$$$$
Murad Age Spot and Pigment Lightening Gel	$$$$
NeoStrata Skin Brightening Gel	$$$
Peter Thomas Roth Potent Skin Lightening Gel Complex	$$$$
Shiseido White Lucent Concentrated Brightening Serum	$$$$$

Rejuvenating Masks

Almay 15 Minute Facial	$
Bliss Triple Oxygen Instant Energizing Mask	$$$
Boscia Moisture Replenishing Mask	$$$
Chantecaille Jasmine and Lily Healing Mask	$$$
ReVive Masque de Glaise	$$$$$

Lip Conditioners

Aquaphor Ointment	$
Aveeno Essential Moisture Lip Conditioner SPF 15	$
Blistex Lip Infusion SPF 15	$
NeoStrata Lip Conditioner SPF 15	$

INTRODUCTION

"Combining what we have seen in our clinical experience with information from psychological studies . . ." "1997 Body Image Survey Results," *Psychology Today* January/February 1997; "Sex Difference in Judgments of Physical Attractiveness: A Social Relations Analysis," *PSBS*, vol. 29, No. 3 (March 2003): 325–35; "Beauty Is As Beauty Does: Body Image and Self-Esteem of Beauty Pageant Contestants" *Journal of Eating and Weight Disorders*, Vol. 3 (September 8, 2003): 231–37; "Peri- and Postmenopausal Changes—Body Awareness, Sexuality, and Self-Image of the Middle-Aged and Older Woman," *Zentralbl Gynakol*, 1225(6) (June 2003): 202–8; "On Models and Vases: Body Dissatisfaction and Proneness to Social Comparison," *Journal of Personality and Social Psychology*, 92(1) (January 2007):106–18.

CHAPTER 1

"Beauty is a universal part of human experience . . ." Nancy Etcoff, *Survival of the Prettiest*, (New York: Anchor Books, 2000), 24.

"According to analysts at Goldman Sachs, worldwide spending on beauty products . . ." Nwe Nwe Yin, "Beauty Industry Undergoing a Facelift," *Myanmar Times*, September 22 28, 2003.

"Brazil now has nine hundred thousand Avon ladies . . ." "The Beauty Business," *The Economist*, May 22, 2003.

"In a 2001 study at Massachusetts General Hospital . . ." I. Aharon, N. Etcoff, D. Ariely et al., "Beautiful Faces Have Variable Reward Value: fMRI and Behavioral Evidence," *Neuron*, Vol. 32 (November 8, 2001): 537–51.

"A 2007 study by researchers at the University of California . . ." Roger Dobson, "Beautiful People Earn 12% More Than Ugly Bettys," *The Independent*, August 12, 2007.

"Psychologist Judith Langlois performed an experiment . . ." Brad Lemley, "Do You Love This Face?" *Discover*, February 1, 2000.

"Evolutionary psychologist Satoshi Kanazawa, of the London School of Economics . . ." Alan S. Miller, Ph.D., Satoshi Kanazawa, Ph.D., "Ten Politically Incorrect Truths About Human Nature," *Psychology Today*, July/August 2007.

"Tall men with high social status have more male offspring . . ." Satoshi Kanazawa, Ph.D., "Big and Tall Parents Have More Sons: Further Generalizations of the Trivers-Willard Hypothesis," *Journal of Theoretical Biology*, vol. 235–34, (August 21, 2005): 583–90.

"In one study, twenty undergraduates rated fifty high school yearbook photos . . ." Joshua J. A. Henderson and Jeremy M. Anglin, "Facial Attractiveness Predicts Longevity," *Evolution and Human Behavior*, Vol. 24-5, (September 2003): 351–56.

"In a massive study of thirty-seven cultures from tribal to modern . . ." D. Buss, M. Abbott, A. Angleitner, et al., "International Preferences in Selecting Mates," *Journal of Cross-Cultural Psychology*, vol. 21-1 (1990): 5–47.

" . . . psychologists videotaped people as they entered a room and introduced themselves." Carlin Flora, "The Beguiling Truth About Beauty," *Psychology Today*, May/June 2006.

"The absence of flaw in beauty is itself a flaw." Havelock Ellis, *Impressions and Comments* (Charleston, SC: BiblioBazaar, 2007), 114.

CHAPTER 2

"As described by John Koo and Andrew Lebwohl in *American Family Physician* . . ." John Koo and Andrew Lebwohl, "Psychodermatology: The Mind and Skin Connection," *American Family Physician*, December 1, 2001.

"UC Davis psychologist Richard Robins attests in *Psychology Today* . . ." Carlin Flora, "The Beguiling Truth About Beauty," *Psychology Today*, May/June 2006.

"The Dutch medical ethicist Medard T. Hilhorst writes that a person's attractiveness . . ." Medard T. Hilhorst, "Physical Beauty: Only Skin Deep?" *Medicine, Healthcare and Philosophy*, Vol.5-1 (March, 2002): 11–21.

CHAPTER 3

" . . .a group of Canadian media researchers generated a computer model . . ." Media Awareness Network, www.media-awareness.ca/english/issues/stereo typing/women_and_girls/women_beauty.cfm

CHAPTER 4

"Humanistic psychology, a field founded by Dr. Abraham Maslow . . ." Abraham H. Maslow, *Farther Reaches of Human Nature*, (New York: Penguin Group USA, 1993).

"According to a 2007 survey by the Pew Research Center . . ." Paul Taylor, Cary Funk, April Clark, "Fewer Mothers Prefer Full-Time Work," Pew Research Center, July 12, 2007.

"A 2007 World Health Organization study published in *Lancet* . . ." S. Moussavi, S. Chatterji, E. Verdes et al., "Depression, chronic diseases, and decrements in health: results from the World Health Surveys," *The Lancet*, Vol 370-9590 (September 8, 2007): 851–58.

"A Dutch study revealed that exercising outdoors . . ." Catharine Paddock, "Green Walking Beats The Blues, New Study Recommends Ecotherapy for Depression," *Medical News Today*, May 14, 2007.

" . . .in a 2004 study at a college in the Southeast, the sight of the color green . . ." Naz Kaya and Helen H. Epps, "Relationship Between Color and Emotion: A Study of College Students," *College Student Journal*, September, 2004.

"In his research, Seligman found that optimistic people . . ." Martin E. Seligman, *Learned Optimism*, (New York: Vintage Books, 2006).

CHAPTER 5

"As Yvonne Antelle wrote in *How to Catch and Hold a Man* . . ." Yvonne Antelle, *How to Catch and Hold a Man* (New York: Essandess Special Editions, 1967).

"If it weren't, U.S. consumers wouldn't be projected to spend $54 billion . . ." "Overweight Consumers and the Future of Food and Drinks," Datamonitor, March 2007.

"The National Institutes of Health's recommendation is to incorporate balance exercises . . ." "Structured Exercise Program May Enhance Seniors' Physical Functioning," National Institute on Aging, www.nih.gov., November 17, 2006.

"You'll strengthen your quads, hamstrings, and abs and burn calories . . ." Laura Berman, Ph.D., "Want to get healthy? Have sex," www.secretsistersociety.com/intimacy.html.

"Twenty-two percent of Americans are getting less sleep . . ." T. Balkin, G. Belenky, C. Drake et al., *2008 Sleep in America Poll*, National Sleep Foundation, March 3, 2008.

"Recommended Health Screenings and Vaccinations . . ." "Preventive Screening Tests and Immunizations," U.S. Department of Health and Human Services, www.4women.gov/screeningcharts.

"Among women over age sixty, the rate of sexually transmitted diseases is rising." Jean Weiss, "Even Grandmas Get STDs," MSN Health and Fitness, health. msn.com/womens-health/articlepage.aspx?cp-documentid=100172026.

"Studies show that regular exercise helps the memory center form . . ." Gretchen Reynolds, "Lobes of Steel," *New York Times*, August 19, 2007.

"Researchers at the University of Arkansas found that men and women . . ." "Study: Better Fitness Means Better Sex," Dye Hard Science, ABC News, abcnews.go.com/Technology/DyeHard/story?id=561491, March 9, 2005.

CHAPTER 6

"As David M. Buss writes in *The Evolution of Desire* . . ." David M. Buss, *The Evolution of Desire* (New York: Basic Books, 2003): 110.

"People with this condition (which is thought to affect 1 to 2 percent of the population) . . ." Rachel Nowak, Cosmetic Surgery Special: When Looks Can Kill," *New Scientist*, October 19, 2006.

"Researchers have found that patients with BDD have a decreased ability . . ." Ulrike Buhlmann, Nancy L. Etcoff, and Sabine Wilhelm, "Emotion Recognition Bias for Contempt and Anger in Body Dysmorphic Disorder," *Journal of Psychiatric Research*, Vol. 40-2 (March 2006): 105–11.

"A woman who doesn't wear perfume has no future." Coco Chanel, quotation, *New York Herald Tribune*, October 18, 1964

" . . .people respond positively to symmetry and averageness . . ." Diane M. Beck, Mark A. Pinsk, and Sabine Kastner, "Symmetry Perception in Humans and Macaques," *Trends in Cognitive Sciences*, Vol. 9-9 (September 2005): 405–6

CHAPTER 7

"The brain has what are called 'mirror neurons,' areas that read and reflect . . ." Sandra Blakeslee, "Cells That Read Minds," *The New York Times*, January 10, 2006.

"Remember the research showing that beautiful people earn more money and get breaks from the legal system?" David B. Sarwer, Leanne Magee, and Vicki Clark, "Physical Appearance and Cosmetic Medical Treatments: Physiological and Socio-Cultural Influences," *Journal of Cosmetic Dermatology*, Vol. 2-1 (January 2003): 29–39.

"Women appear to have more mirror neurons than men." Eric Weiner, "Why Women Read More Than Men," NPR Online, www. npr.org/templates/story/story.php?storyId=14175229 September 5, 2007.

"Ronald Riggio, Ph.D., a psychology professor at Claremont McKenna College . . ." Mark Greer, "The Science of Savoir Faire," *Monitor on Psychology*, January 2005: 28.

"Frank Bernieri, Ph.D., of Oregon State University . . ." Greer, 29–30.

"Being in close contact sets off the brain's hormonal reward circuitry . . ." Gale Berkowitz, "UCLA Study on Friendship Among Women," Women's Circles, http://womenscircles.us/WomensCircles/tabid/36/articleType/ArticleView/articleId/46/UCLA-Study-on-Friendship-Among-Women.aspx, July 6, 2007.

"Even more intriguing, Chris Dunkel Schetter, a UCLA psychologist . . ." P. Feldman, C. Dunkel-Schetter, and C. Sandman et al., "Maternal Social Support Predicts Birth Weight and Fetal Growth in Human Pregnancy," *Psychosomatic Medicine*, Vol. 62 (2000): 715–25.

CHAPTER 8

"A 2005 survey by *Allure* magazine called "The Allure of Beauty Study . . ." *Allure*, September 2005.

" . . .a British insurance company surveyed women in the United Kingdom . . ." "Britons Spend a Lifetime $54,000 on Shoes," *Iran Daily*, August 8, 2005.

"A 2007 *Consumer Reports* issue reviewed antiaging creams . . ." Nancy Metcalf, "Wrinkles—What Treatments Work?" *Consumer Reports*, January 2007.

"According to the American Lung Association, smoking-related disease . . ." "Quit Smoking," American Lung Association, www.lungusa.org/site/pp.asp?c=dvLUK9O0E&b=33484.

CHAPTER 9

"In a speech in 1959, John F. Kennedy said . . ." Remarks at the Convocation of the United Negro College Fund, Indianapolis, Indiana, April 12, 1959.

" . . .affects the lives of about twelve million U.S. women each year . . ." National Institute of Mental Health, "Unpublished Epidemiological Catchment Area Analyses," 1999.

"Studies have shown psychotherapy to be effective for lifting depression." "Psychotherapy's Effectiveness in Depression Is Demonstrated by Two Studies Using High and Low Therapy Doses," Medical News Today, www.medical newstoday.com/articles/69417.php, May 1, 2007.

" . . .studies in England suggest that couples' counseling . . ." Edward M. Waring, et al., "A Pilot Study of Marital Therapy as a Treatment for Depression," *American Journal of Family Therapy*, Vo. 23-1 (spring 1995): 3–10.

"Anxiety disorders also affect millions of American women . . ." "Statistics and Facts About Anxiety Disorders," Anxiety Disorders Association of America.

"In a provocative study, women suffering from depression experienced a reduction . . ." Eric Finzi, M.D., Ph.D., "Treating Depression with Botox, *Journal of Dermatologic Surgery*, Vol. 32 (May 2006): 645–50.

CHAPTER 10

"More than eleven million cosmetic surgical procedures were performed in the United States in 2006 . . ." "11.5 Million Cosmetic Procedures in 2006," American Society for Aesthetic Plastic Surgery, March 9, 2007.

"Plastic surgery became popular in this country after World War I . . ." Karol A. Gutowski, "A Plastic Story: A Short History of Plastic Surgery," *JAMA* Vol. 293 (April 2005): 1798.

"One large U.S. study revealed that 70 percent of married men . . ." E. J. Mundell, "Does Size Matter? Most Romantic Partners Say 'No'," The Sexual Health Network, sexualhealth.e-healthsource.com/?p=news1&id=525946, May 27, 2005.

CHAPTER 11

"Okinawans are among the longest-lived people on Earth . . ." Dan Buettner, "Secrets to Longevity," *National Geographic*, November 2005.

Books We Love

About Face: A Plastic Surgeon's 4-Step Nonsurgical Program for Younger, Beautiful Skin by Gregory Bays Brown, M.D.

Absolute Beauty by Pratima Raichur with Marian Cohn

Age Proof Your Body by Elizabeth Somer, M.A., RD

Allure: Confessions of a Beauty Editor by Linda Wells

Away with Wrinkles by Nicholas Lowe, M.D.

Basic Black: The Essential Guide for Getting Ahead at Work (and in Life) by Cathie Black

Beautiful Skin of Color by Jeanine Downie, M.D.; Fran Cook-Bolden, M.D.; with Barbara Nevins Taylor

Don't Go to the Cosmetic Counter Without Me by Paula Begoun

Don't Sweat the Small Stuff by Richard Carlson, Ph.D.

Emotional Intelligence by Daniel Goleman

Feeling Good: The New Mood Therapy by David D. Burns, M.D.

Fit and Sexy for Life by Kathy Kaehler

Getting the Love You Want by Harville Hendrix, Ph.D.

I Feel Bad About My Neck by Nora Ephron

InStyle—Getting Gorgeous by the editors of *InStyle*

Learned Optimism by Martin Seligman, Ph.D.

Light Years Younger by David Goldberg, M.D., and Eva M. Herriott, Ph.D.

Living Beauty by Bobbi Brown

The Memory Prescription by Gary Small, M.D., with Gigi Vorgan

The Millionaire Zone by Jennifer Openshaw

O's Guide to Life by the editors of *O, the Oprah Magazine*

The 7 Habits of Highly Effective People by Stephen R. Covey

The South Beach Diet by Arthur Agatston, M.D.

Survival of the Prettiest by Nancy Etcoff

What You Wear Can Change Your Life by Trinny Woodall and Susannah Constantine

You: The Owner's Manual by Michael Roizen, M.D., and Mehmet Oz, M.D.

Younger Next Year for Women by Chris Crowley and Henry S. Lodge, M.D.

WEBSITES WE LOVE

beautyandthebrain.com

drluftman.com

psychiatry.med.miami.edu

thebeautyprescription.com

HEALTH

American Academy of Dermatology—aad.org

American Psychiatric Association—psych.org

Anxiety Disorders Association of America—adaa.org

everydayhealth.com

kathykaehlerfitness.com

The National Women's Health Information Center—4women.gov

oprah.com

realwomensfitness.com

Skin Cancer Foundation—skincancer.org

thinkpink.com

women.webmd.com

womenfitness.net

Women's Health magazine—womenshealthmag.com

FOOD

allrecipes.com

bonappetit.com

cookinglight.com

eatingwell.com

epicurious.com

foodnetwork.com

gourmet.com

myrecipes.com

Skin Care

beauty.ivillage.com

doctorgoodskin.com

healthyskinportal.com

iqbeauty.com

makeup.com

Skin and Cancer Associates Center for Cosmetic Enhancement—scacce.com

skincareguide.com

smartskincare.com

therapeutix.com

Medical

cosmeticsurgery.com

ginamarcusdmd.com

healthgrades.com

medicinenet.com

physicianreports.com

Physicians' Research Network—prn.org

Stress Management

mindtools.com

stressmanagementtips.com

Also see sites listed under "Health."

INDEX

Acne, 30, 31, 117, 136, 138, 140, 145, 146, 150, 196, 240, 250, 251–52, 268–69

Adversity, 215–16, 239. *See also* Stress

Aerobic exercise, 106, 200

Aestheticians, 140, 161, 196, 261

Affirmations, 93, 208, 209

Age/Aging
  acting your age, 180–82, 187
  change and, 67
  life beauty plan and, 196–204
  menopause, 105–6, 138, 256
  skin and, 139–42

Alcohol, 91, 115, 129, 141, 198, 201, 231–32, 238

Anxiety, 38, 227–28

Attractiveness, 15–17, 43

Barbie, cult of, 47–49

Beauty. *See also* Inner beauty; Life Beauty Plan; Outer beauty
  attractiveness, 15–17, 43
  evolving, 13–15
  innate, 11–13
  as a journey, 271–72
  magnetism, 15, 16–17, 32

Beauty and the Brain Rx
  clearing cobwebs, 187–88
  cosmetic priorities, 168
  empowerment, 25–26

essentials, 71–72
foundation for beauty, 44–45
optimism, 95–96
self-defeating patterns, 263
sleep, 125
smoking cessation, 212–13
stress management, 239–40
tanning products, 262

Beauty Boosters
  eye care, 60
  eye contact, 152
  firm boundaries, 89
  listening skills, 177
  mind makeover, 113
  passions, 226
  peels, 198
  positive thinking, 10
  precautions against infections, 253
  water and healthy foods, 37

Beauty-Brain Loop
  beauty bullets, 44
  becoming a blue light special, 29, 31
  confidence paradox, 40–42
  defined, 31–33, 38–39
  discipline, empowerment, and optimism, 28–29
  inner beauty and, 32, 33, 39, 76–77
  mastering, 22, 35–38, 40, 269–71

outer beauty and, 32, 33, 130–33,
    270
  working the, 42–43, 237
Beauty Buddies
  bonding over lunch, 7
  businesswomen, 192–93
  getaways for, 51–52
  inspiring women, 171–72
  marathon runners, 217
  political activists, 101
  sharing stories about, 273
  sisters, 78
  traveling buddies, 130–31
Beauty Bullets
  beauty that's skin deep and
    deeper, 24–25
  Beauty-Brain Loop, 44
  cosmetic medicine, 261–62
  health, 124–25
  inner beauty, 95
  outer beauty, 167
  staying beautiful, 211
Beauty Busters
  bold changes, 19
  change and age, 67
  crying, 229
  fear as motivator, 39
  fighting, 181
  self-esteem and beauty, 91
  skin-care products, 204
  suntans, 118–19
  telltale signs of surgery, 259
  wrinkles and dryness, 145
Beauty Pearls
  eyebrows, 162
  financial success, 220
  grace and poise, 21
  hair care, 156
  inner beauty, 48, 87
  lighting, 257

recipe for skin treatment, 151
safe cosmetics, 141
smiles, 41
three key factors, 206
three tips for looking better,
    34–35
Beauty Prescription Quiz
  beauty bullets, 70–71
  environment section, 63–66
  goal of, 52
  health section, 57–60
  inner beauty section, 54–57
  meaning of, 68–70
  outer beauty section, 61–63
  rating your attitude, 53
  scoring, 66–68
Beauty Story topics
  baby blues, 106
  battered women, 247
  cancer survivors, 175
  depression, 82
  hirsutism, 137
  lip enhancement, 195
  liposuction, 56
  makeovers after neglect, 12–13
  mourning process, 222
  stress and skin disorders, 30–31
Body dysmorphic disorder (BDD),
    133–34
Botox, 144, 145, 175, 197, 199,
    200, 202, 203, 208, 237, 242,
    253–54, 259

Cellulite, 258, 262
Charisma, 179–80
Clothes and fashion, 165–67
Collagen, 138, 139, 140, 144, 145,
    146, 200, 204, 251, 255, 256
Combination skin, 136, 147, 148,
    149, 150

Confidence paradox, 40–42
Cosmetic procedures
    beauty bullets, 261–62
    dermatologists and, 248–49
    for hair-related problems, 137,
        256–57
    as lifelong change, 245–48
    for lines and wrinkles, 252–56
    noninvasive procedures, 249–52
    plastic surgeons and, 259–61
    realistic expectations and, 244–45
    right reasons for, 242–43
    spider veins, cellulite, and,
        257–59
Cosmetics
    advice on, 159–63
    safety of, 141
    saving on, 207
    storage of, 187
    updating, 34–35
Crying, 229

Dark circles, 60
Dental care, 121, 157–59
Depression
    appearance and, 38, 237
    cognitive distortions and,
        239–40
    Janine's story, 82
    meditation and, 117
    overall health and, 86
    postpartum, 106
    signs of, 129, 226
    sleep patterns and, 125
    treatment for, 225–27
Dermatologists, 140, 161, 196, 207,
    248–49, 261
Diet. *See* Nutrition tips
Dieting, yo-yo, 100–101, 141
Disagreements, healthy, 181

Dove campaign, 27–28
Dry skin, 136, 147, 148, 149, 150,
    197

Evolving beauty, 13–15
Exercise, 104–9, 212, 238
Eye care, 60, 254
Eye contact, 152
Eye cream, 60, 148, 149, 150
Eye exam, 121
Eyebrows, 162
Eyelid lift, 201, 202, 254

Face-lifts, 201, 202–3, 245, 251
Faith lift, 17–20, 22, 25

Goals, achievable, 93
Gratitude, 94, 211

Hair care, 35, 153–57
Hair-related problems, 137, 256–57
Health, 97, 98–100, 132. *See also*
    Wellness
Health care, 104, 119–22
Health section of quiz, 57–60
Hirsutism, 137, 256–57
Humor, 93

Innate beauty, 11–13
Inner beauty
    beauty bullets, 95
    calamity and, 224–25
    defined, 32, 76–77
    fitness, self-awareness, and, 90–92
    having it all, 81–83
    living inside out, 83–87
    mental tools for, 92–95
    optimism for, 87–90, 95–96
    quiz section on, 54–57
    self-esteem and, 76–77, 79, 270

Snow White versus wicked queen,
79–80
strengths, 92
stress and, 131
Inner Beauty Plan, 208–11
Intense pulse light (IPL), 145, 201,
202, 203, 250, 252, 256

Jewelry, 164–65

Kindness, 93, 210, 230, 236

Lasers, 146, 250–51, 256
Life Beauty Plan
ages fifty to sixty, 201–2
ages forty to fifty, 199–201
ages sixty and beyond, 202–4
ages thirty to forty, 197–99
ages twenty to thirty, 196–97
money for, 194–96, 204–5,
207–8
Lighting, 257
Lip enhancement, 195, 255
Liposuction, 258–59
Listening, active, 177, 180

Magnetism, 15, 16–17, 32
Makeup
advice, 159–63
safety of, 141
shopping for, 207
storage of, 187
updating, 34–35
Media detox, 185–86
Melanoma, 118–19, 197
Menopause, 105–6, 138, 256
Mental health problems. *See also*
Stress
anxiety, 38, 125, 227–28

cognitive distortions, 239–40
depression, 38, 82, 86, 106, 117,
125, 129, 225–27, 237
Mental health professionals,
232–34, 239
Mental tools for daily living,
92–95
Metacognition, 83
Microdermabrasion, 144, 147, 148,
149, 150, 160, 197, 199, 250,
252, 261
Mind makeover, 113
Mirror neurons, 175, 176, 231
Moments, magic, 186, 209
Money issues, 194–205, 207–8, 220

Nail care, 150–53
Nutrition tips, 37, 104, 109–14,
141, 143, 145, 153, 204, 238

Obesity, 100–102
Oily skin, 136, 147, 148, 149, 150
Optimism, 87–90, 95–96
Osteoporosis, 105, 107
Outer beauty
beauty and brain Rx, 168
in Beauty-Brain Loop, 130–33,
270
beauty bullets, 167
clothing, 165–67
distorted self and, 133–35
hair, 153–57
jewelry, 164–65
makeup, 159–63
nails, 150–53
perfume, 163–64
quiz section on, 61–63
skin, 135–50
stress and, 237–38
teeth, 121, 157–59

Passions, pursuing your, 94–95
Peels, chemical, 144–45, 160, 197, 198, 249–50, 252, 261
Perfume, 163–64
Plastic surgeons, 259–61
Plastic surgery. *See* Cosmetic procedures
Posture, 124

Quiz, Beauty Prescription
    beauty bullets, 70–71
    environment section, 63–66
    goal of, 52
    health section, 57–60
    inner beauty section, 54–57
    meaning of, 68–70
    outer beauty section, 61–63
    rating your attitude, 53
    scoring, 66–68

Relationships, importance of, 86, 183–85, 266–67
Retinoids, 72, 144, 147, 148, 149, 150, 200, 204
Risks, taking, 93, 210
Rosacea, 20–21, 117, 145, 150, 198, 252
Rowland, Cynthia, 192–93

S-lift, defined, 202–3
Self-actualization, 76–77
Self-care, 84, 218–19, 237–38
Self-doubt, 37
Self-esteem, 76–77, 79, 83, 91, 122, 131, 270
Self-talk, positive, 86, 90, 209
Sex, 105, 108, 119, 124
Skin
    anti-aging options for, 139–46
    five types of, 136
    sun-damaged, 34, 118–19, 139–40, 142–43, 251–52
    three layers of, 138–39
Skin care
    daily regimen, 146–50, 160–61
    prescription, 71–72
    teaching teens about, 268–69
Sleep, 104, 114–116, 125, 231, 236
Smoking, 140, 157, 208, 212–13, 239
Spider veins, 257–58
Spirituality, 89–90, 236
Strength, beauty and, 234–37
Strength training, 107, 200
Strengths, emphasizing, 92
Stress
    crisis and emotions, 224–25
    effects of, 131, 140–41, 154, 240
    management, 86, 104, 116–17, 239–40
    self-care and, 218–19, 237–38
    skin disorders and, 30–31, 240
Stressful periods (transitions), 216, 218
Sun damage, 34, 118–19, 139–40, 142–43, 251–52
Sunscreen, 72, 118–19, 142–43, 147, 148, 149, 156, 160, 207, 211
Support networks, 266–67. *See also* Beauty Buddies

Tanning products, 262
Teeth, 121, 157–59

Vaccinations and health screenings, 120–21
Vampire strategy, 142
Varicose veins, 258

Water, 37, 44, 111, 143, 207
Weight, obsession with, 100–102
Wellness
    components of, 104, 270
    exercise, 104–9, 212, 238
    glow of, 103–4
    health care, 104, 119–22
    nutrition, 37, 104, 109–14, 141,
        143, 153, 238
    sleep, 104, 114–116, 125, 231,
        236
    stress management, 104, 116–17

Work and inner beauty, 94
Wrinkles. *See also* Skin
    age and, 197–204
    cosmetic procedures for, 249–56
    moisturizers and, 145
    prevention and treatment options
        for, 142–46, 149
    skin-care products and, 204
    sun damage and, 34, 118–19,
        139–40, 142–43, 251–52

Yo-yo dieting, 100–101, 141